INFANTS, TODDLERS, AND FAMILIES

INFANTS, TODDLERS, AND FAMILIES

A Framework for Support and Intervention

Martha Farrell Erickson
Karen Kurz-Riemer

THE GUILFORD PRESS
New York   London

© 1999 The Guilford Press
A Division of Guilford Publications, Inc.
72 Spring Street, New York, NY 10012
http://www.guilford.com

Printed in the United States of America

This book is printed on acid-free paper.

Last digit is print number: 9 8 7 6 5 4 3 2 1

Library of Congress Cataloging-in-Publication Data

Erickson, Martha Farrell.
    Infants, toddlers, and families : a framework for support and
intervention / Martha Farrell Erickson, Karen Kurz-Riemer.
       p.   cm.
    Includes bibliographical references and index.
    ISBN 1-57230-487-1 (hardcover)
    1. Infants—Services for—United States.   2. Toddlers—Services
for—United States.   3. Family services—United States.   4. Child
welfare—United States.   5. Socially handicapped children—Services
for—United States.   I. Kurz-Riemer, Karen.   II. Title.
HV741.E77 1999
362.7'083'20973—dc21   99-32761
                                                                 CIP

To our children, Ryan and Erin Erickson and Jess and Liz Riemer, who years ago enriched and expanded our knowledge of infant and toddler development. They continue to be our best teachers on this most important journey of parenthood.

About the Authors

Martha Farrell Erickson, PhD, is Director of the Children, Youth and Family Consortium at the University of Minnesota, where she links research to practice and policy for the well-being of children and families. A developmental psychologist, she specializes in parent–child attachment, child abuse prevention, and community-based approaches for strengthening families. With research colleague Byron Egeland, Dr. Erickson developed the STEEP program (Steps Toward Effective, Enjoyable Parenting) and continues to do related speaking and consulting throughout the United States and abroad. The author of numerous scholarly publications, Dr. Erickson also writes a syndicated parenting column, "Growing Concerns," and appears weekly as the parenting expert for KARE-TV. She is the mother of two young adult children.

Karen Kurz-Riemer, MEd, is a family education consultant, writer, and trainer, based in Minneapolis. A former childhood teacher and adminis-trator, she played a leading role in coordinating the early development of Minnesota's Early Childhood Family Education (ECFE) program from six pilot programs in the mid-1970s to a statewide program that serves nearly 300,000 parents and children each year. She has assisted the Min-nesota Department of Children, Families, and Learning as ECFE expands its statewide activity with families of infants and toddlers. The focus of her work is the well-being of children and families at all points in the life cycle, beginning with the newborn period. She is the parent of an adult stepson and two teenage daughters.

Preface

What do you think of when you hear the term "early intervention"? Whom do you picture as the recipients of services? What is the nature of these services, and whom do you see delivering them and in what setting?

Since the passage of Public Law 99-457 in 1986, "early intervention" to many people has meant special education services to children with identifiable handicapping conditions. Certainly, that is one important segment of the field of early intervention; nevertheless, it is still only one aspect. In this book, we use the term "early intervention" to describe a much larger domain of services. Early intervention as discussed in this book encompasses many programs—often in health care, mental health, or human service settings—aimed at infants and toddlers who are considered to be at risk due to some condition of birth or circumstance (e.g., premature infants, children in poverty, infants born to parents who are chemically dependent or mentally ill).

The early intervention principles and strategies discussed throughout this volume will also be useful in parenting programs for the general public. Even healthy children born into stable, financially secure, well-functioning families can benefit from programs that provide their parents with emotional support, accurate information about child development, and a chance to explore their own underlying attitudes and beliefs about children and relationships. Taking a very broad perspective, early intervention also might be viewed as encompassing the field of child care. Not only do child care providers have a direct impact on the children in their care, but they are also in a powerful position to support and encourage parents as the major facilitators of a child's optimal development.

The grouping together of such a broad array of so-called early intervention services is supported by the striking convergence of findings from studies of various populations—children with disabilities, so-called high-risk children and families, and children in the general population. The factors associated with positive child outcomes, and strategies for helping families promote those good outcomes, appear to be much the same across varied groups and settings.

Let's consider, for example, three families who might be recipients of some kind of early intervention services:

Family 1: Marcia and Doug's second child, Lisa, was diagnosed with Down syndrome at birth. In the 6 weeks since Lisa's birth, Marcia has been exhausted and depressed, weeping often, sleeping poorly at night, but dozing often during the day. Two-year-old Jason is aggressive toward his new baby sister and has begun to throw frequent temper tantrums, further exhausting Marcia. Doug has thrown himself into his work, coming home late most nights. He often sits in the nursery in the dark, worrying about the future as he watches Lisa sleeping.

Family 2: Judy is a 17-year-old high school dropout who recently gave birth to her first child, Danny. Judy is not sure who Danny's father is, and she has been estranged from her own parents since dropping out of school and running away. Throughout her pregnancy she moved from place to place, staying with acquaintances until they would kick her out because she couldn't help with expenses. Judy professes to be thrilled to have a cute little baby all her own and seems eager for information on his development. She expresses high aspirations for the kind of person Danny will grow up to be and vows that "no one's gonna mess him up like people did to me."

Family 3: Tammy is a precocious toddler who walked at 8 months and spoke in complete sentences by the time she was 17 months old. Her parents, Rick and Sandy, put her name on the waiting list of a prestigious private school shortly after Tammy was born. Each day when Rick and Sandy return from work they do flash card drills with Tammy, working on letters and numbers, and they are proud that she already counts to 10. But they have recently been exasperated that Tammy seems more interested in chewing on the flash cards or throwing them on the floor and laughing. They suspect it is because the child care provider is spoiling Tammy and letting her get away with too much, and they wonder if they should change child care arrangements.

What are the needs and strengths in each of these three unique families? What factors are likely to facilitate each child's optimal development? What are some potential barriers to the competence and well-being of the children and families? What might early interventionists do to support each of these families and promote each child's healthy development? How likely are these families to obtain the information and support they need?

The first family would be eligible in most states for early intervention services because of their new baby's diagnosis of Down syndrome. Depending on where they live, the second family might be eligible for services because of the risk status associated with adolescent parenthood. The third family would be unlikely to receive any kind of service unless they sought out a parenting class on their own. Yet all three families are ripe for some type of early, supportive intervention. The three families differ markedly in terms of life circumstances and the special challenges they face. However, when we look beyond a superficial description of their situations, common issues become apparent: developing appropriate expectations for child behavior; remaining responsive to the needs of the child in the face of stress and frustration; finding adequate social support and opportunities to share and explore feelings about parenting; and examining values and beliefs about child rearing. This is early intervention—a broad domain indeed!

As programs evolve to respond to the needs of diverse families such as these, early intervention professionals from various disciplines face new challenges, in terms of both the developmental and familial problems to which they must respond and the demands to collaborate with each other in these efforts. Each discipline brings special knowledge and skills to this venture. Parent educators bring knowledge of effective child-rearing practices and skill in providing adult education, while health care professionals contribute awareness of the impact of health practices on the overall development of the child. Early childhood educators offer the ability to create learning environments that facilitate the young child's development in all domains. Psychologists have a background in cognitive and emotional development and specialized skills in assessment, while special educators bring understanding of various disabilities and specialized teaching strategies. Social workers contribute an understanding of how the broader familial and community environment can be strengthened to promote the young child's well-being. Speech and language clinicians provide an understanding of the role that communication plays in the child's development, and physical and occupational therapists offer unique perspectives on the child's physical adaptation to the people and objects in the environment.

Despite the distinct emphasis of each separate discipline, there are—and, we believe, should be—more similarities than differences in what the various professionals do with young children and their families. It is the similarities of function and orientation that we address here. In writing this book we have drawn from a broad body of recent literature related to early intervention strategies, as well as the research and practice in which we have been involved over the years. And, perhaps most important of all, we have incorporated information and insights gleaned from professionals and practitioners we have met through consulting and speaking around the country—nurses in rural Minnesota, social workers in New York City, school psychologists in Oklahoma, special educators and early interventionists in Washington state, early childhood educators in Hawaii—whose stories echo strikingly similar themes. Their experiences have affirmed and enriched the knowledge derived from our own study and practice.

This book does not attempt to provide all the answers or to be a "cookbook" of early childhood intervention practices. Rather, it provides a framework for intervention, identifying common themes and integrating theory and research relevant to promoting optimal development for infants and toddlers. (An extensive annotated bibliography at the end of the book directs service providers to useful hands-on resources for practice.)

Specifically, in Chapters 1 and 2, we present background information on the historic roots of early intervention and current directions for practice. In Chapters 3–5, we discuss critical themes and strategies for working with families with young children, covering issues related to parenting behavior, beliefs and feelings, and social support. Throughout all five chapters, we address ways to adapt those strategies with diverse populations, including families of different cultural backgrounds, families whose children have special needs, and parents who face challenges such as mental illness or chemical dependency.

An underlying principle throughout the book is that the most effective interventions occur when service providers free themselves from narrowly prescribed professional roles. Experience and research strongly suggest that flexible, client-centered approaches are what work, and those approaches rarely line up perfectly with a template of any one professional's job description. At the heart of effective intervention is the relationship between service provider and client, a relationship too often impeded by organizational constraints. This book, then, is written with the hope that it will challenge and inspire leaders in the field of early intervention to stretch the systems in which they work, to find ways to let their services be shaped by the needs and strengths of the child and family more than by job descriptions. Whatever your role in the early intervention enterprise, we hope you will find new insights and information, as well as affirmation of what you already have discovered through your work with young children and their families.

Acknowledgments

With deep respect and gratitude, we salute the many lively children, valiant parents, and dedicated colleagues whose lives and work informed this book. You are too many to name, but we thank you.

Special thanks to Dr. Jacqueline Schakel of Anchorage, Alaska, for her significant contributions to our review of history and best practices in early intervention; Connie Blasing of the Children, Youth and Family Consortium, who knows that the devil is in the details; and the independent booksellers—Oleanna Books of Minneapolis, and Redleaf Press and Hungry Mind Bookstore of St. Paul—who generously offered access to their rich book collections.

And thanks, of course, to Ron Erickson and Rick Riemer for their love and encouragement as we brought this project to completion.

Contents

ONE

Early Intervention: Where We've Been and Where We're Going

In a moving article published January 1, 1992, in the Minneapolis Star-Tribune, *Kristine M. Holmgren describes a home for "profoundly retarded" children where her mother worked in 1965: "They were the babies and toddlers of the wealthy; children who were privileged to not be sent to [the public institutions]. Their families paid dearly to lodge their child in a crib in the lovely home near the lake. . . . [I]t was stuffed with military issue cribs. The kids lived in those beds, row by row. They ranged from 6 weeks to 15 years. . . . The children were smaller than the cribs that jailed them, flat on their backs. Rules were that they were to be taken from their cribs only if sick or dead. . . . My mother fed them a diet of pabulum and powdered milk, mixed with heavy vitamins and laxatives. She changed their diapers, laundered their T-shirts, booties, and linen. She followed the strict orders to never pick them up; never hold them. . . . " (p. 19A)*

When we first began working with children in the mid- to late 1960s, "early intervention" was not even in our professional vocabulary. State hospitals were crowded with so-called mentally handicapped children who had languished there from an early age, often fulfilling society's expectation that they were capable of learning little or nothing. Families who allowed their children with disabilities to remain at home usually received no formal support or training in how to meet the child's special needs. A parent who had concerns that an infant's development was off-

1

track commonly was advised to "wait and see if the baby outgrows it," only to wait and see months or years later that the child was, indeed, disabled in some way and perhaps had developed secondary emotional or cognitive difficulties as a result of the lack of understanding of the primary disability.

Thirty years ago, a toddler living in abject poverty and lacking appropriate stimulation and opportunities for exploration had little hope of intervention until entering kindergarten, at which time he or she was already far behind age mates in social skills and academic readiness. Even in kindergarten there were few resources to help him succeed.

Although we still have far to go, the field of early intervention has come a long way in those 30 years. The importance of the early months of life in setting the stage for later adjustment and success is now well known, based on an accumulation of research and experience. Early intervention is enabling children to overcome many obstacles that block their optimal development and helping families to adapt to the individual needs of their children. In recent years, we as a society seem to have arrived at (or, at least, are moving steadily toward) a collective belief that "it is never too soon." Whether a child is born with Down syndrome; born to a teenage mother with little education; or born into a high-achieving, affluent family, there is a strong impetus to provide experiences in the first months and years of life that will enable that child to adapt successfully.

In this chapter we (1) review briefly some of the historical background of early intervention (Where We've Been), tracing the trends in research and practice that have brought us to where we are today; and (2) identify current trends and future directions for interventions that are built on a solid foundation of knowledge about what really matters for infants and toddlers and their families (Where We're Going).

WHERE WE'VE BEEN

Over the past 30 years, three large bodies of theory, research, and clinical findings have converged, providing a persuasive (although sometimes inconclusive) argument for early intervention and exerting an ongoing influence on the nature of early intervention services. These three major bodies of work include (1) basic developmental theory and research on the influence of early experiences on a child's subsequent development, (2) documentation of the impact of early intervention on the later achievement and adjustment of children who are disadvantaged due to poverty and related stressors, and (3) findings on the effects of early intervention on the ongoing adaptation and learning of children with disabilities. Information gleaned from these endeavors provided incentive for the development of a wide range of educational, medical, and human service programs for infants and young children with varied needs and backgrounds and, in 1986, inspired a federal legislative and monetary incentive (Public Law 99-457) to serve children with disabilities from birth to school age. Because we believe it is important to examine where we have been in order to begin to understand where we are going and why, let's review some of the achievements and failures of the past that have brought us to this juncture in early intervention.

Basic Theory and Research in Child Development

The 20th-century began without serious attention to the study of child development and the factors that influence its course for better or for worse. In the 1920s, however, as a result of a growing interest in the effects of heredity and environment on human development, psychologists began to consider the relative importance of "nature versus nurture." The debate that ensued continues to affect practice in early intervention to this day. Representing the two extremes in this debate were Gesell and Watson. Every early interventionist needs to be familiar with the "nature versus nurture" debate to understand current beliefs about children's development and how it is influenced through early intervention.

NATURE VERSUS NURTURE

Gesell espoused an ardent belief in the biologically based unfolding of behavior as a child matured, regardless of experience. Through observational studies of normally developing children, babies who were born prematurely or suffered perinatal injuries, and children with Down syndrome, Gesell carefully documented sequences of development from infancy through the school years (e.g., Gesell, 1925; Gesell & Thompson, 1934). These sequences were considered to be very predictable. By documenting them in detail, Gesell and his colleagues hoped to be able to predict future development in children based on these biologically predetermined sequences of growth. In his view, early intervention was rather useless; experience could not alter what was biologically determined.

This biological view was adapted by researchers in the 1950s who explored the link between perinatal insult (caused by difficult births) and later developmental problems (Lilienfeld & Parkhurst, 1951; Lilienfeld & Pasamanick, 1954). Their explanation for later disorders, which came to be called the "continuum of reproductive casualty," traced a direct line from perinatal events to developmental outcomes. In other words, given a certain type and severity of perinatal injury or problem, one could predict how an individual child would develop.

This maturational perspective on development and its emphasis on a child's biological "nature" continue to influence practice in early intervention. Many practitioners still use Gesell's well-documented developmental sequences for determining what is "normal" or not for a child at a particular age. In fact, these sequences provided the basis for many instruments used in developmental assessment (including the Bayley Scales of Infant Development; Bayley, 1969, 1992). When, for example, a speech and language specialist discourages impatient parents from seeking articulation therapy for a 2-year-old who can't pronounce the letters R and L, the specialist is acting on an informed understanding of the typical oral–motor development of young children and the inadvisability of trying to push children beyond the current development of their biological capabilities. On the other hand, when well-meaning professionals recommend delaying entrance into kindergarten for a child solely because a test indicates that the child is not "maturationally ready" to benefit from school, that may represent too strict an interpretation of the maturational perspective that fails to take nurture into account. In that case, further assessment would be needed to determine other possible explanations for the child's performance, including, for example, lack of opportunity for learning or a cognitive or a behavior problem with deeper roots than simple immaturity.

Representing a view opposing Gesell in the nature–nurture debate, Watson (1928) argued that, except in cases of severe brain damage, environment and experience (aspects of nurture) were the major influences on development. This position, sometimes characterized as the "blank slate" perspective, assumed that parents were largely responsible for rearing competent, well-adjusted children despite the children's genetic make-up. Many early behaviorists, in a logical extension of Watson's position, advocated for programs that would provide children with the stimulation lacking in their normal daily environment.

Because of strong beliefs in the primacy of inherited and biological characteristics at the time Watson first propounded his theories, this point of view was not well received in scientific circles until much later. A now-famous study by Skeels and Dye (1939) was one of the first to show the positive impact on development of a change in the quality of a child's environment, yet it received very little positive attention at the time. In this controversial study, 13 children under the age of 3 were taken from an orphanage where they received only routine attention to physical needs and minimal contact with adults. These children were placed on a ward of a hospital serving mentally retarded young women.

In addition, researchers provided toys and educational materials. You may well imagine the attention these infants and toddlers received from these female residents, who were probably quite deprived of stimulation themselves! The children received a considerable amount of stimulation and affection unlike anything they had experienced in the orphanage. When IQ scores were obtained on this experimental group and compared to the IQ scores of children who remained in the orphanage, striking differences were noted. Children placed in the young adult ward and provided with stimulation showed an average *gain* of 27.5 IQ points; children left behind in the orphanage showed an average *loss* of 26.2 points.

If these striking findings had been taken seriously, this study might have been the beginning of the early intervention movement and a focus on nurture. But because of the strength of scientists' belief in the importance of nature at the time, the findings were disregarded. In fact, the study's results were criticized and ridiculed by some of the most influential psychologists of the time, including Goodenough and McNemar (Hunt, 1961). For example, McNemar refuted the Skeels and Dye (1939) findings, stating that the IQ results could be explained entirely by the fact that the orphanage children were not used to adult attention and thus were not as cooperative in the testing session as the experimental children. He concluded that the findings failed to support the environmental hypothesis and were entirely consistent with a hereditarian view. Although we would certainly agree with him now that testing conditions and children's previous experiences influence their scores on formal tests, it is unlikely that they would explain so large a difference. And, in fact, little by little, in spite of biases in the scientific community toward the nature viewpoint, new evidence began to accumulate that would eventually tip the balance in the debate to a focus on nurture.

Much of this early evidence came from experimental studies of lower animals. For example, in the early years of his career, Hunt (1961) showed that rats deprived of consistent feeding were more likely to hoard food in adult life, even when well fed as adults. Interestingly, Hunt went on from animal studies to theories of child development and became one of the most articulate spokesmen for the view that experience and environment have a strong effect on children's intelligence (Hunt, 1961).

Another animal researcher, Harlow (1958), documented the impact of maternal deprivation in his study of rhesus monkeys separated from their mothers at birth and raised in isolation for the first 6 months of life. These monkeys displayed unusual behaviors such as crouching in a corner of their cage, rocking, and grasping themselves. Later in life, these motherless monkeys had problems in social interaction including displays of extreme fear and aggression, atypical responses to sexual approach, and, in the few cases in which females mated successfully, abuse and neglect of their offspring. During infancy, when given a choice between a wire "mother" holding a bottle of milk or a soft cloth "mother" with no bottle, Harlow's monkeys preferred the cloth mother most of the time, even though it did not provide nourishment. They also showed a preference for surrogate mothers that were warm and for ones that rocked rather than remaining still.

Scientists at the time questioned if results of animal studies could be applied to humans; however, evidence from studies of children also began to accumulate. In a classic study published in 1945, Spitz reported on an investigation of the development of infants living in an orphanage (similar to the one from which Skeels and Dye [1939] removed their 13 subjects and typical of orphanages at the time), where they received basic physical care but only minimal personal attention from caregivers and few or no opportunities for emotional involvement with others. At 1 year of age, these babies had become extremely passive, rarely crying or smiling and making no attempt to speak. Not surprisingly, on tests of mental functioning, most of the infants performed in the retarded range. Fifteen years after publication of this study, the tide had turned in favor of nurture.

Hunt (1961) cited Spitz's studies as being most influential in convincing people that intelligence is not genetically fixed and that mothering is crucial during the first year of life. Other strong support came from studies by Goldfarb (1943, 1955) and Provence and Lipton (1962). Hunt's 1961 book, *Intelligence and Experience*, reviewed the accumulated evidence from these and other studies and concluded, "In light of these considerations it appears that the counsel from experts on child rearing during the third and much of the fourth decades of the 20th century to let children be while they grow and to avoid excessive stimulation, was highly unfortunate" (p. 362). It is a sign of how much thinking has changed over the years that these findings were greeted with surprise back in the late 1950s, whereas now, reading this, you're probably thinking, "Well, of course!"

There were others writing in the mid-20th century from the psychoanalytic perspective whose work continues to be influential in early intervention to this day. Bowlby (1951) received support from the World Health Organization to investigate the effects of homelessness and maternal deprivation on children's mental health. His focus on the universal importance of the mother–child relationship and his later conceptualizations of the term "attachment" (Bowlby, 1969) have become well known in early intervention circles; they provide one cornerstone for much of what we believe is important in early intervention today.

TRANSACTIONAL VIEWS

Reviewing the evidence on the powerful effects of caregiver–child relationships on a child's development, and believing as we do now in the importance of early intervention, you might find yourself tempted to discard the nature perspective altogether just as scientists prior to 1940 discarded the nurture perspective. After all, we can't do much about a child's nature, and, from the early intervention perspective, nurture is what we might be able to alter. But researchers attempting to prove one view to the exclusion of the other have always come up short. We should be looking instead at the roles of nature *and* nurture. Biology (including a child's genetic make-up and physical characteristics) determines the capacity for a broad range of possible behaviors and outcomes. Environment influences the path of development taken from among all the possibilities.

For example, nearly all human infants are born with the capacity to learn to communicate, but whether or not they develop oral speech, what language they use, and the accuracy of grammar and syntax all depend on what they experience in their environment. As another example, a child with severe orthopedic problems is unlikely to become a world champion ice skater; however, there are many possible futures open to this child and environmental factors will play a major role in determining which one becomes reality.

Appreciating the effects of both biological and environmental factors on development is not enough by itself. It's also important to look at the way they influence each other. In the 1970s, this concept was articulated in what was to become a classic discussion of the "transactions" among biological, social, and environmental influences on development. Sameroff and Chandler's transactional model (1975) offered a contrast to the early notion of the "continuum of reproductive casualty" discussed previously, in which children identified as having had complications at birth were expected to exhibit problems in later development. Sameroff and Chandler's "continuum of *caretaking* casualty" illustrated how the impact of a child's biological strengths and vulnerabilities could be either buffered or enhanced by positive or negative environmental factors.

One helpful way to conceptualize this transactional model is to picture a noncompetitive tennis match with the child's biological nature on one side and the environmental and social factors in a child's life on the other (Wohlwill, 1973). From the time the first serve is made, what happens on one side of the net depends on what just happened on the other. If the players are not well matched, with one player being much stronger than the other, the strong player's serves and volleys will be not be returned skillfully most of the time. But how they are returned depends not just on the skill of the player returning the ball but also on how it was served by the other player. To keep the game going, one player may have to adjust to the skill and style of the other.

So it is with transactions between caregivers and children. The prospect of handling a tiny infant, no matter how alert and responsive, may strike fear in the heart of a new mother or father who is unprepared for parenthood. The response might be to withdraw from interaction with the infant, and the infant may, in turn, become less and less responsive. Yet, if the parent overcomes the fear and responds to the infant's sociable nature, the infant is likely to continue a positive interaction. In this transaction, the parent is able to *nurture* the child's sociable *nature*.

Support for this model came from a now famous and oft-cited study known as the Kauai Longitudinal Study (Werner, Bierman, & French, 1971). A total of almost 700 children born on the island of Kauai, Hawaii, were studied from the prenatal period on to adulthood (Werner, 1987, 1989; Werner & Smith, 1977, 1982). These children came from both affluent and impoverished families. The study showed that one of three children developed learning or behavior problems by age 18 and that most of these children with poor outcomes had experienced multiple risks, including complications at birth, poverty, family instability, and parental psychopathology. Although these findings might lead you to interpret that biological and/or environmental risks *do* predict poor outcomes directly, the fact is that 10% of all the children in the study had experienced these same risk factors before the age of 2 and still developed into competent, well-adjusted young adults (Werner, 1990). We know now that there may be protective factors both within the child and/or within the child's environment that transact to produce favorable outcomes in spite of early risk.

Building on the tradition of a transactional view of development, recent research on brain development has brought the concepts of nature and nurture together in new and provocative ways. Thanks to technological advances that allow neuroscientists to see inside the infant's brain, we are learning how experience (nurture) affects the very structure (nature) of the growing child's brain. These new findings further strengthen the case for early intervention and support for infants and their caregivers (Shore, 1997).

Basic child development research continues to contribute valuable information to the field of intervention, and recent findings from this basic research will be discussed further in later chapters. Now, however, we turn to the large body of research on the effects of preschool intervention with disadvantaged children, our second body of important research for early intervention.

Early Intervention and Disadvantaged Children

HEAD START

Another branch of research and experience that has had a major impact on early intervention is the compensatory education movement for disadvantaged children, best known through *Project Head Start*. Although Montessori in Rome and the MacMillan sisters in London (Peterson, 1987) had already created successful nursery schools for preschool-age children growing up in the slums in the early 1900s, it wasn't until the 1960s that compensatory education programs were developed in the United States. As a result of the civil rights movement and the exposure of poverty conditions within a seemingly affluent American society by the Kennedy and Johnson Administrations, Project Head Start was conceived as a means for helping children break out of the cycle of poverty. Started in 1965, Head Start was designed to be a way to prepare children for success in school, not only through education but also through improvements in nutrition, health care, social and emotional development, and parental attitudes toward and involvement in the education of their children. Because success in school was most often defined as high achievement and cognitive development, those who sought to assess the value of the Head Start experience for a child most often measured its effects on children's scores on IQ and achievement tests.

Although several studies were conducted to answer the question "Is Head Start effective?", conflicting answers were obtained. Early reports (between 1965 and 1968) were positive and optimistic, showing what seemed to be immediate positive effects on children in terms of increases in IQ scores and school achievement in kindergarten and first grade. But authors of a well-publicized study by the Westinghouse Learning Corporation in 1969 questioned the lasting value of Head Start into the early grades of school, although they emphasized the positive effects of the program on parents. Unfortunately, the lack of positive results on children's cognitive growth led many policy makers to brand Head Start a failure (see Zigler & Valentine, 1979, for an account of Head Start's history and relevant evaluations). However, two important recommendations of the Westinghouse report had powerful and long-lasting effects on the early intervention community: (1) To be most effective, intervention with disadvantaged children and their families should begin in infancy; and (2) *parents* are the key to a child's future success and should be assisted in helping their own children.

Later studies of Head Start's effectiveness suggested that previous reports of negative results were overstated and misguided. Although indeed, many Head Start children did not maintain into third grade the cognitive gains they made initially, some showed a "sleeper effect" that appeared in grade 5.

The Head Start model also was applied to some programs for infants and home-based programs for preschoolers, although these programs never reached the scope of Head Start. *Parent and Child Centers* applied the Head Start model to children from birth to age 3 in an attempt to prevent the negative impact of poverty at an earlier age. Many of these programs still continue today. Whereas Head Start services were typically delivered in center-based programs, *Home Start* attempted to provide such services to families in their own homes through use of home visitors. As Head Start has grown during the last several years, programs have evolved to include both home- and center-based components.

OTHER COMPENSATORY PROGRAMS

A discussion of where we've been in early intervention would not be complete without mention of the Ypsilanti Perry Preschool Project (also known as High/Scope). Initiated in the Ypsilanti, Michigan, public schools in 1962 (even before the beginning of Head Start), this study has documented the educational, social, and economic benefits of early intervention with economically disadvantaged children (Berrueta-Clement, Schweinhart, Barnett, Epstein, & Weikart, 1984; Schweinhart & Weikart, 1980). Through this program, researchers were able to follow 123 children from low-income black families far beyond their preschool experience in the Perry Program and to compare them to a control group of children who did not receive preschool intervention. Results showed that children from the preschool performed better on achievement tests throughout the school years and were less likely to be placed in special education. There were noneducational benefits reported as well, lasting into early adulthood—greater likelihood of pursuing higher education, higher employment rates, less crime and delinquency, and fewer early pregnancies.

This was also one of the first projects to attempt to evaluate the monetary benefits of early intervention. Through careful cost–benefit analysis, it was estimated that the preschool intervention provided by the Perry Program, although expensive to operate, resulted in long-term savings through reduced costs for special education programs, higher earning power of graduates, and savings from reduced crime (Barnett, 1985). Savings per participant in the program were figured to be about $15,000 or about a 243% return on the original dollar investment.

Although the findings of the Perry Preschool Program have been controversial (for a review, see Farran, 1990), they continue to be commonly cited as evidence for the effectiveness of a particular kind of early intervention program in improving the lives of children. A summary of this and other early intervention studies with disadvantaged preschool children is provided in a report entitled, "Lasting Effects of Early Education" by Lazar and Darlington (1982).

Perhaps of more interest to those of us who work with infants are the interventions with disadvantaged children that begin prior to the age of 36 months. Several important studies commenced in the 1960s or early 1970s, with results reported in the late 1970s and early 1980s. As with the early preschool studies, these projects followed children considered at risk for school problems, usually those from families of low socioeconomic status (SES). Unlike the preschool studies, however, these projects usually reflected a home-based model of intervention rather than a center-based model, although some compared home- versus center-based models. Typically, in the home-based model, an intervener came to the home with materials for promoting cognitive and language development through play. Parents were taught to use these materials for stimulating the development of their infants and toddlers—the emphasis was on producing changes in the child, not in the parent.

Results of the most often-cited studies with disadvantaged infants and toddlers were mixed. Some showed that home visiting had no positive effects on children; others showed that home visits were better than no intervention at all but not as effective as center-based care; still others showed children's cognitive development improved by either a home visit program or a center-based program. Classic studies in this category include the Carolina Abecedarian Project (e.g., Ramey, Bryant, Sparling, & Wasik, 1985; Ramey & Campbell, 1984), Gray's Home Visit Program (Gray & Ruttle, 1980), the Family Development Research Program at Syracuse (Honig & Lally, 1982), and the Mailman Center Projects (Field, Widmayer, Greenberg, & Stoller, 1982).

BRONFENBRENNER'S REVIEW AND CONCLUSIONS

Another important review of research was a report entitled, "Is Early Intervention Effective?" by Bronfenbrenner (1975). He reviewed research findings from early intervention programs carried out in preschool settings outside the child's home and interventions conducted in a child's home through visits from an early interventionist. Because Bronfenbrenner's conclusions have so strongly influenced the design of subsequent early intervention programs, they are presented in some detail here.

His 1975 report suggested that preschool programs and home-based tutoring programs benefited children in terms of cognitive gains, but that these gains were not maintained after termination of the intervention. It is important to note that he found differences in the way particular groups of children responded to intervention. Children from very poor socioeconomic backgrounds appeared to gain least from early intervention and to lose ground more quickly than children in families with better circumstances. Interventions that focused on the parent as well as the child produced longer-lasting gains. Bronfenbrenner pointed out that interventions that were designed to improve parent–child interactions had the greatest benefits; they nurtured positive reciprocal interactions that lasted beyond the intervention, and they had a positive effect on siblings as well. The timing of these parent–child interventions seemed to make a difference, too, with greater gains for programs started for children and their parents before the children reached age 2. Participation in a parent–child program prior to entering preschool also seemed to enhance the preschool experience. Bronfenbrenner concluded that the family is the most economical and effective system for supporting the child's development. Without the involvement of family, intervention is likely to fail, and any positive effects are likely to be short-lived.

An important aspect of Bronfenbrenner's writing then and since has been his emphasis on "systems" (Bronfenbrenner, 1979). His "ecological" model takes into account the many formal and informal social units and networks (e.g., the immediate family, the extended family, networks of friends and neighbors, churches, agencies, and policy-making groups) that affect what happens in a child's life and the way these social networks are interdependent. This ecological perspective considers how events in one unit may affect other units. For example, how fully a family is able to take advantage of an early intervention may be affected by needs of siblings, opinions of aunts and uncles, neighborhood support, agency policies, and so on. Bronfenbrenner pointed out that many families live in such dire and impoverished circumstances that they are unable to participate in early intervention programs because just living from day to day takes so much of their energy (Bronfenbrenner, 1975). As we shall discuss, these ideas serve as a basis for much of the early intervention that occurs today, not only for at-risk children, but also for children with disabilities.

Early Intervention and Children with Disabilities

EARLY STUDIES

Research on the impact of early intervention on children with disabilities has a history going back to the late 1940s when Kirk designed preschool programs for children with mental retardation who lived in an institution. As was true with basic developmental research and with research on the effectiveness of intervention with disadvantaged children, these early studies focused chiefly on cognitive outcomes. Kirk found that compared to a control group receiving no intervention, these children had an average gain of 10 IQ points as opposed to a loss of 6.5 IQ points (Kirk, 1958). Whereas none of the control group left the institution, almost half of the experimental children did so and were placed in foster homes.

Studies of children with Down syndrome (Hanson, 1985; Hayden & Haring, 1976, 1977; Oelwein, Fewell, & Pruess, 1985) were quite common among early investigations of the effectiveness of intervention with children who experienced disabilities, perhaps because this syndrome could be readily identified. Research in the late 1960s and early 1970s had shown that when children with Down syndrome were reared at home and did not receive early intervention, there were declines in measures of cognitive development (Birch & Cornwell, 1969; Dicks-Mireaux, 1972). Intervention research demonstrated that participants in early education programs manifested developmental milestones earlier and maintained higher rates of development into the elementary school years. Similar findings were obtained with infants who had delays in neurological development and hearing impairments (e.g., Horton, 1974).

The benefits of early intervention for blind babies also were demonstrated in one of the first early intervention studies to focus on social rather than cognitive outcomes (Fraiberg, Smith, & Adelson, 1969). This research showed that a 3-year home intervention program in which parents were taught to teach and handle their blind infants was effective in increasing and enhancing the social behavior of these infants. As you will see in later chapters, this and other work by Fraiberg has greatly influenced the techniques currently used to assist parents of infants with disabilities in interacting with their babies.

An excellent summary of intervention studies on children with disabilities was provided in Farran's (1990) "decade review" in the *Handbook of Early Childhood Intervention*. He notes that some studies involved somewhat homogeneous populations of children (e.g., children with Down syndrome), whereas others involved a wide variety of children, including those with developmental delays of unknown cause. Ages of entry into intervention, length of intervention, extent of parent involvement in intervention, and measures of change in the children all varied. Some researchers reported long-term follow-up data, but typically this did not occur. Most investigations reported data gathered on children for less than a year. Because of these discrepancies and problems, it was difficult to draw definite conclusions from the early studies. In spite of this, however, several key people in the field of special education began to lobby for increased services at a very early age to children with disabilities. Their efforts resulted in new legislation that would dramatically increase interest in early intervention.

FEDERAL LEGISLATION AND RELATED INITIATIVES

Just as the compensatory education movement for disadvantaged preschools and infants got its biggest boost from a government-sponsored program (Project Head Start), the first major impetus for the field of early intervention for children with disabilities also came through federal legislation. In 1968, Public Law 90-538 (the Handicapped Children's Early Education Assistance Act) provided money for developing model programs to serve children with disabilities. These projects, known as *Handicapped Children's Early Education Projects* (HCEEP) or *First Chance* projects, were designed to try out a variety of intervention procedures and disseminate the most effective ones across the country. At about the same time, the Bureau of Education for the Handicapped and the Division of Maternal and Child Health began to award grants to universities for developing training programs that would prepare personnel to work with young children with disabilities. In 1973, the Council for Exceptional Children, an organization representing special educators, started a special division (the Division for Early Childhood) for people concerned with providing services to children younger than school age.

In 1976, the Battelle Institute published a summary of the evaluation of 32 HCEEP model intervention programs (Stock et al., 1976). Unlike earlier evaluation studies, this one used a pre- and posttest measure designed to test children's development in five developmental domains: motor skills, cognition, communication, personal–social development, and adaptive behavior. The evaluation also included a parent survey to assess parent perceptions of changes in their children, family involvement in the early intervention program, and parent satisfaction with the program. Results suggested that the early interventions had a significant effect in four of the five developmental domains. Both home- and center-based programs were effective, but home-based programs produced larger effects. The parent survey provided important confirmation of what parents of children with disabilities had been expressing informally to early interventionists—parent satisfaction was high and parents benefited by gaining knowledge on how to work with their children and insights into realistic expectations for their children's development.

At this time, there were still no broad-based services for children with disabilities who were younger than age 5. By providing monetary incentives, Public Law 94-142, the Education for All Handicapped Children Act (passed in 1975 and later renamed the Individuals with Disabilities Education Act [IDEA]), encouraged states to serve children as young as age 3 through the public schools. As a number of states developed these early education programs for 3- to 5-year-olds with disabilities during the late 1970s, a few states extended these services to children even younger. As interest in infant intervention grew, the National Center for Clinical Infant Programs was created to boost awareness of the needs of infants with disabilities and those who were considered at risk for such disabilities.(Now known as "Zero to Three," this still is a major center for linking research to practice.) By 1985, seven states had mandatory services for children with disabilities from birth onward, even though there was no federal mandate for such services.

A few other influential studies published around this time deserve mention because of the impetus they gave to the early childhood special education movement. Although early interventionists and parents of children with disabilities may have been convinced about the importance of early intervention already, policymakers needed evidence that such programs could be cost effective. The Colorado State Department of Education (McNulty, Smith, & Soper, 1984) and Roy Littlejohn Associates (Reaves & Burns, 1982) documented the savings involved in early intervention by showing that if children with disabilities received services in the early years, they were less likely to need special services in elementary school. Reports of the Early Childhood Research Institute at Utah State University (Casto & Mastropieri, 1986; Casto, White, & Taylor, 1983) attempted to summarize almost 450 studies of early intervention and documented the short-term effects of early intervention, although these studies raised questions about how lasting those effects were. As we will discuss in the next chapter, these studies all had flaws and can be criticized. No study suggested that every type of early intervention works for every type of child; but the important effect of this accumulating body of evidence was that as a whole it presented a convincing argument for early intervention for children with disabilities.

The climax of this drama was the passage in 1986 of Public Law 99-457 (reauthorized in 1991 as Public Law 102-119). Through the efforts of many organizations and lobbyists, this law was proposed, passed, and signed into law in a very short time. Lobbying efforts on the part of early interventionists and parents were so intense that at one point White House operators reportedly were answering the telephone, "Are you calling about the early intervention bill?" (B. Smith, personal communication, June 12, 1992). Although the law did not mandate nationwide early intervention services, the monetary incentives were so strong and the arguments so persuasive that every state indicated the intention of putting such services into effect. A brief summary of the part of this legislation that affects services to infants and toddlers (Part H) is provided here.

Public Law 99-457, Part H. This legislation appropriated funds to states for the planning, development, and implementation of services to "handicapped infants and toddlers." This includes children who are identified as "developmentally delayed" as defined by each state, children who have conditions that typically result in such delays, and (at the discretion of each state) children who are at risk of substantial developmental delay. States have defined eligible children in many different ways; it is important to refer to your state's regulations for information about those children your state recognizes as eligible.

The law required that each child be provided a multidisciplinary assessment and that a written Individualized Family Service Plan (IFSP) be developed by a multidisciplinary team and the parents. One person is designated to coordinate the services of each child and family. The IFSP must contain (1) a statement of the child's present levels of development in cognitive, communication, social–emotional, motor, and adaptive domains; (2) a statement of the family's strengths and needs relating to enhancing their child's development; (3) a statement of planned outcomes for the child and family; (4) the criteria, procedures, and timelines for determining progress; (5) the specific services necessary to meet the needs of the child and family; (6) the initiation dates and expected duration of the services; (7) the name of the service coordinator; and (8) procedures for transition from early intervention into the preschool program. It is important to note that although this law contained many of the same provisions as the earlier Public Law 94-142, the emphasis was not strictly "educational," but more broadly included mental health and prevention services for the family and child. Among the services that can be written into the IFSP and funded through this legislation are family training, social skills training, counseling, parent consultation, and home visits.

Further support for these early intervention programs came with the IDEA Amendments of 1991 (Public Law 102-119), which reauthorized the Part H Program. This legislation refined the language of the previous law, increased funding for early intervention services, emphasized the importance of providing services in "natural environments," gave parents the right to refuse some services while accepting others, and directed states to adopt policies that ensure involvement of traditionally underserved groups such as minority, low-income, rural, and Native American families. And in 1997, amendments to IDEA further expanded the focus of the infant and toddler programs (now renamed "Part C") to include the development of a system of coordinated services for infants and toddlers with disabilities. Although advocates had hoped for a permanent reauthorization of early intervention services, the new legislation extends the program only to the year 2002.

Early Intervention and "Normal" Infants and Toddlers

Almost all publicly funded programs have eligibility requirements, and early intervention programs are no exception. To receive services under Public Law 99-457, children must fit a state's definition of "developmentally delayed" or "at risk." To participate in Head Start or similarly funded programs, families must meet income guidelines and other requirements. What in the history of early intervention has been done for "normal" or "typically developing" infants and their families?

Traditionally, "normal" infants and their families have not been seen as needing intervention, so few programs were developed for them. The first programs that were developed were designed for parents who wished to accelerate their infant's development. One program developer who capitalized on the desires of members of the "baby boom" generation to maximize their children's intellectual potential was Doman. Through books such as *How to Teach Your Baby to Read* (1964), *Teach Your Baby Math* (1979), and *How to Multiply your Baby's Intelligence* (1983), and through his Better Baby Institute, Doman encouraged parents to push their infants to develop their maximum brain power. Among his most often-discussed and controversial methods was to expose infants as young as 3 months to flashcards with pictures of letters, numbers, shapes, colors, and even famous historical figures and works of art. The popularity of these programs serves as a good example of how practice is often based on shaky or nonexistent research evidence. Although many parents who could afford it invested in Better Baby Institute seminars and materials and participated enthusiastically (participation was so widespread as to generate a cover story in *Newsweek* [Langway, Jackson, Zabarsky, Shirley, & Whitmore, 1983]), there were no published studies of the program's effectiveness and most child development experts at the time described many aspects of the program as useless and perhaps even harmful.

But there were also less controversial, though underfunded and relatively invisible, programs for normally developing children. The Parent and Child Center programs, begun in the early 1970s, represented a new emphasis on parent education to improve the lives of infants from low-income families. While these programs were large, federally funded demonstration projects, at the same time a number of grass-roots, community-based programs with local funding were also started. Weiss and Halpern (1991) list the *Avance* program started in Houston in 1973; *Family Focus* in Evanston, Illinois; and the Minnesota *Early Childhood Family Education* programs as examples. These grass-roots efforts, because of their community base, emphasized the role of families rather than professionals in providing the direct stimulation that would produce good outcomes in children. Now several states have gone a step beyond providing programs solely to families at risk and are assisting local agencies in funding voluntary primary prevention to *all* families, as is done in Minnesota's Early Childhood Family Education program. Many such programs are being implemented under the auspices of Healthy Families America, an initiative of the Chicago-based Prevent Child Abuse America. These programs are built on a philosophy that every parent and caregiver can benefit from learning nurturant parenting skills and that such learning results in making the family environment a better place for human development (Weiss & Halpern, 1991).

As with the movements in child development research, at-risk programs, and programs for children with disabilities, the trend in programs for the "typical" family has been away from sole emphasis on encouraging cognitive gains in children to a more global emphasis on overall adjustment for the child and family. It is clear that in today's world, with its high stress and diminished social supports, all parents can use support and education. Perhaps by making such services universally available, we also can make them more appealing (and less stigmatizing) to the high-risk families who may need them most.

WHERE WE'RE GOING

Having discussed what has already happened in this brief history of early intervention, we have arrived at the present, with the ongoing challenges of implementing Public Law 99-457 (and its subsequent amendments), intervening with at-risk families, and providing supportive services for the general population of infants and their families. Considering where we were at midcentury, we've come very far in the last 40 to 50 years! Let's review some of the trends, current issues, challenges, opportunities, and potential pitfalls facing us in early intervention. This will provide us a framework for the interventions we propose throughout the rest of this book.

Keeping the "Early" in Early Intervention

As knowledge about child development has advanced, it has become apparent that in many, if not all, cases, earlier is better. An accumulation of research in neuropsychology suggests that early in development, the neural tissue is very receptive to environmental experiences (Anastasiow, 1990; Greenough & Green, 1981; Shore, 1997) and that child development is more plastic in the early years. For example, neuroscientists have shown that a baby's experiences with caregivers lay down the "auditory maps" for language; strengthen the neural connections that enable the child eventually to develop complex, logical reasoning; and shape the parts of the brain that regulate emotion and control impulses.

We also have evidence that interventions that begin prenatally can have a significant impact on the future lives of children and their families (e.g., Barnard, Morisset, & Spieker, 1993; Olds, Henderson, Tatelbaum, & Chamberlain, 1986, 1988; Olds & Kitzman, 1990). Pregnancy is a time for mental and emotional preparation for the tasks of parenting, a time to examine beliefs and expectations and build or strengthen social supports. And, of course, throughout pregnancy the mother's physical health, nutritional status, and emotional well-being have a direct effect on the health of the growing baby.

If we were able to cast financial considerations aside, many of us would agree that it is better to start programs earlier rather than later and to work in a proactive, preventive way rather than intervening after problems occur (Upshur, 1990). (Of course, research on what works best when and with whom will need to be a continued focus.) Consequently, a trend in early intervention is to start work as early as possible in the life of a child with identified disabilities and risk factors, or, in many cases, to work with prospective parents even before their child is born.

Evolving beyond Focusing Only on Cognitive Stimulation

In early research and intervention studies, services to infants and preschoolers were a downward extension of models used with older populations. Because of this, the focus was often on increasing children's IQ and later school achievement. In reviewing the early research, we learned how measured gains in IQ were often lost when intervention was discontinued, and we saw a gradual shift from a focus on cognitive outcomes to a broader set of outcomes. In current practice, there is a recognition not only of the importance of other domains of development, but also of the interrelatedness of these domains. Even if we wanted to focus exclusively on cognitive outcomes, it would be impossible. In infancy and early childhood, cognition, language, motor skills, adaptive skills, and social–emotional functioning are all important and inextricably intertwined. Furthermore, influencing a young child's attitudes and motivation, as well as the support networks that nurture and encourage the child, may ultimately be the most effective way to promote the child's subsequent achievement.

Becoming Noncategorical and Individualized

Models for serving older children, particularly those with disabilities, traditionally classified children into categories and applied intervention accordingly. Thus there were separate interventions for children with Down syndrome, those who were blind, those who were hearing impaired, those who had speech impairments, those who were disadvantaged by poverty, and so on. Current practice recognizes that interventions may work across categories and that programs for children should be based on their individual needs and the needs of their families, rather than on the particular category into which they may be classified. In most early intervention programs today, you will find many kinds of children being served together.

For example, young children with disabilities, once served almost entirely in segregated and categorical programs, are now viewed as needing to be fully integrated with normally developing children. In addition, rather than a preplanned program of activities to be offered to all participants regardless of needs, current interventions are typically designed to meet the needs of the child and family and arrange for the type and level of involvement that is most appropriate.

Our challenge will be to select, design, and modify interventions so that they meet the unique situation of each child and family. This will require assessments that consider all relevant aspects of the child and family and awareness of the limitations of each intervention approach that we may have in our repertoire. It also will require cooperation among agencies and services, as no one program will be able to meet all the individual needs of each child and family.

Moving into a Context Focus

In the early years of research and intervention with young children, the focus of intervention programs was either the child or the parent in isolation. For example, special education programs for young children with disabilities were often downward extensions of programs for older children in the schools and thus were designed to provide stimulation and remediation solely to the child. Progress and program success were measured by assessing the child's cognitive growth. Research into autism, for another example, focused on the role of the mother's personality in "causing" this problem, and psychotherapy for the mother was viewed as the appropriate treatment.

Now, because of all we have learned, early intervention and assessment of its effectiveness focus on the child in the context of the family and the family in the context of the larger community. We no longer attempt to intervene with a child without giving major consideration to family strengths, needs, and wishes. We no longer focus on changing a parent's style of dealing with a child's behavior without also considering the characteristics the child brings to the interaction.

A major challenge for the future in early intervention will be to gain a better understanding of the context in which families operate. As Gallagher (1990) pointed out in his review of the effectiveness of family intervention, we know that negative factors in a family's environment may affect the family's ability to benefit from early intervention. We also are discovering the unintended consequences to families that may accompany our well-meaning attempts to intervene. And we are just beginning to explore and understand the cultural differences that may affect a family's response to early intervention and the importance of recognizing the degree of acculturation to the dominant culture of each family with whom we work (García Coll & Meyer, 1993; Vincent, Salisbury, Strain, McCormick, & Tessier, 1990). These are challenges indeed for early interventionists!

Focusing on Strengths More Than Deficits

In the past, many early intervention programs have been based on a medical model in which the challenge is to identify what is wrong and then treat it. Thus programs focused on a child's and a family's deficits and attempted to correct them. As the field of early intervention moves toward a more context-focused model, we not only are considering families, community supports, and cultural influences as important. We are also recognizing that it is critical to understand these contexts as assets to be drawn on to improve a child's chances of benefiting from early intervention. In the past, a focus on what was wrong with the child and family encouraged dependence on early interventionists and programs. We became "experts" or "helpers" to whom families turned for answers. The focus now has shifted to assisting families in drawing on their own strengths and resources for solutions.

Balancing the Needs of the Child with Desires of the Family

This notion sounds easy, but is sometimes a very difficult balance to achieve. As early interventionists have become more involved with children's families and the contexts in which they function, some of us have probably become overzealous in our attempts to help children by helping their families. We have all encountered family members who may not perceive the need for supportive services or who may not have the time, money, transportation, skills, or confidence to access services. There are also families who have been so traumatized and stressed by earlier encounters with "the system" that they do not want any "interference" from outside agencies or may see intervention as an invasion of privacy. Our efforts to involve these families in our well-meaning attempts to see that their children get what they need may only result in resistance and the creation of more barriers between us. A continuing goal for early interventionists is to work on ways to engage families without invading privacy, encouraging overdependence, or putting ourselves in the "expert" role.

Employing Collaboration and the Sharing of Resources

A result of many of the trends and issues we have discussed is that we recognize that simple linear models of intervention don't work. There is no one program that will work to prevent drug and alcohol use in pregnant teens, nor is there a single intervention that will effectively treat developmental delays in children. As we tailor programs to the individual needs of each child and family, we will have to work collaboratively; no one agency can do everything for every child and family. In each individual community, consumers and providers of services will need to collaborate rather than compete to take advantage of scarce financial resources. This also will mean joining together to influence public policy. Our experiences with the passage of Public Law 99-457 show that when agencies and citizens cooperate, much can be accomplished.

How far have we come? Contrast this description of a typical day, excerpted from an interview with a mother of a 2-year-old with severe disabilities, with the vignette at the beginning of the chapter.

> "Christopher and I spend the morning together doing the things that parents and their kids usually do—eating breakfast, dressing, going to the park if it's a nice day. It probably takes us a little longer than normal, but we're used to that. . . . I love having Chris with me in the morning. His smiles are the highlight of my day! . . . In the afternoon, I have to go to work so I drop him off at [the child care center] two blocks away. He is the only child there who doesn't walk, but they've always got him right in the middle of every activity. . . . I've taught them how to read Chris's body language so communication is not usually a problem. There's a woman who comes from the school district to work on other ways of teaching him to communicate. I visit with her at least once a week when I drop him off, and she comes over to our apartment in the morning sometimes. She's been a big help to me—not just with Chris but in a lot of ways. If it wasn't for her, I don't think I would have had the

courage to apply for a job. . . . The adults and the kids at Chris's child care all love him. I'd say he gets more than his share of hugs. . . . "

REFERENCES

Anastasiow, N. J. (1990). Implications of the neurobiological model for early intervention. In S. J. Meisels & J. P. Shonkoff (Eds.), *Handbook of early childhood intervention* (pp. 196–212). New York: Cambridge University Press.

Barnard, K. E., Morisset, C. E., & Spieker, S. (1993). Preventive interventions: Enhancing parent–infant relationships. In C. H. Zeanah, Jr. (Ed.), *Handbook of infant mental health* (pp. 386–401). New York: Guilford Press.

Barnett, W. S. (1985). Benefit–cost analysis of the Perry Preschool Program and its policy implications. *Educational Evaluation and Policy Analysis, 7,* 333–342.

Bayley, N. (1969, 1992). *Bayley Scales of Infant Development.* New York: Psychological Corporation.

Berrueta-Clement, J. R., Schweinhart, L. J., Barnett, W. S., Epstein, A. S., & Weikart, D. P. (1984). *Changed lives: The effects of the Perry Preschool Program on youths through the age 19.* Ypsilanti, MI: High/Scope.

Birch, H., & Cornwell, A. (1969). Psychological and social development in home-reared children with Down syndrome. *American Journal of Mental Deficiency, 74,* 341–350.

Bowlby, J. (1951). *Maternal care and mental health* (World Health Organization Monograph No. 2). Geneva: World Health Organization.

Bowlby, J. (1969). *Attachment and loss: Vol. 1. Attachment.* New York: Basic Books.

Bronfenbrenner, U. (1975). Is early intervention effective? In M. Guttentag & E. L. Struening (Eds.), *Handbook of evaluation research* (Vol. 2, pp. 519–603). Beverly Hills: Sage.

Bronfenbrenner, U. (1979). *The ecology of human development by nature and design.* Cambridge, MA: Harvard University Press.

Casto, G., & Mastropieri, M. A. (1986). The efficacy of early intervention programs: A meta-analysis. *Exceptional Children, 52,* 417–424.

Casto, G., White, K., & Taylor, C. (1983). An early intervention research institute: Studies of efficacy and cost effectiveness of early intervention at Utah State. *Journal of the Division for Early Childhood, 7,* 37–48.

Dicks-Mireaux, M. J. (1972). Mental development of infants with Down syndrome. *American Journal of Mental Deficiency, 77,* 26–32.

Doman, G. (1964). *How to teach your baby to read.* New York: Random House.

Doman, G. (1979). *Teach your baby math.* London: Pan.

Doman, G. (1983). *How to multiply your baby's intelligence.* Philadelphia: Better Baby Press.

Farran, D. C. (1990). Effects of intervention with disadvantaged and disabled children: A decade review. In S. J. Meisels & J. P. Shonkoff (Eds.), *Handbook of early childhood intervention* (pp. 501–538). New York: Cambridge University Press.

Field, T., Widmayer, S., Greenberg, R., & Stoller, S. (1982). Effects of parent training on teenage mothers and their infants. *Pediatrics, 69,* 703–707.

Fraiberg, S., Smith, M., & Adelson, E. (1969). An educational program for blind infants. *Journal of Special Education, 3,* 121–139.

Gallagher, J. J. (1990). The family as a focus for intervention. In S. J. Meisels & J. P. Shonkoff (Eds.), *Handbook of early childhood intervention* (pp. 540–559). New York: Cambridge University Press.

García Coll, C. T., & Meyer, E. C. (1993). The sociocultural context of infant development. In C. H. Zeanah, Jr. (Ed.), *Handbook of infant mental health* (pp. 56–69). New York: Guilford Press.

Gesell, A. (1925). *The mental growth of the preschool child.* New York: Macmillan.

Gesell, A., & Thompson, H. (1934). *Infant behavior: Its genesis and growth.* New York: McGraw-Hill.

Goldfarb, W. (1943). Infant rearing and problem behavior. *American Journal of Orthopsychiatry, 13,* 249–265.

Goldfarb, W. (1955). Emotional and intellectual consequences of psychological deprivation in infancy: A reevaluation. In P. H. Hoch & J. Zubin (Eds.), *Psychopathology of childhood.* New York: Grune & Stratton.

Gray, S., & Ruttle, K. (1980). The Family-Oriented Home Visiting Program: A longitudinal study. *Genetic Psychology Monographs, 102,* 299–316.

Greenough, W. T., & Green, E. J. (1981). Experience and the changing brain. In J. L. McGaugh, J. G. March, & S. B. Kiesler (Eds.), *Aging, biology, and behavior* (pp. 71–91). New York: Academic Press.

Hanson, M. J. (1985). An analysis of the effects of early intervention services for infants and toddlers with moderate and severe handicaps. *Topics in Early Childhood Special Education, 5,* 36–51.

Harlow, H. F. (1958). The nature of love. *American Psychologist, 13,* 673–685.

Hayden, A. H., & Haring, N. G. (1976). Programs for Down's syndrome children at the University of Washington. In T. Tjossem (Ed.), *Intervention strategies for high-risk infants and young children* (pp. 573–608). Baltimore: University Park Press.

Hayden, A. H., & Haring, N. G. (1977). The acceleration and maintenance of developmental gain in Down's syndrome school-age children. In P. Mittler (Ed.), *Research to practice in mental retardation: Care and intervention* (pp. 129–142). Baltimore: University Park Press.

Honig, A., & Lally, R. (1982). The family development research project: A retrospective review. *Early Child Behavior and Care, 10,* 41–62.

Horton, K. B. (1974). Infant intervention and language learning. In R. L. Schiefelbeusch & L. L. Lloyd (Eds.), *Language perspectives: Acquisition, retardation, and intervention* (pp. 211–232). Baltimore: University Park Press.

Hunt, J. M. (1961). *Intelligence and experience.* New York: Ronald Press.

Kirk, S. A. (1958). *Early education of the mentally retarded.* Urbana, IL: University of Illinois Press.

Langway, L., Jackson, T. A., Zabarsky, M., Shirley, D., & Whitmore, J. (1983). Bringing up superbaby. *Newsweek, 101,* 62–68.

Lazar, I., & Darlington, R. (1982). Lasting effects of early education: A report from the Consortium for Longitudinal Studies. *Monographs of the Society for Research in Child Development, 47*(2–3, Serial No. 195).

Lilienfeld, A. M., & Parkhurst, E. (1951). A study of the association of factors of pregnancy and parturition with the development of cerebral palsy: A preliminary report. *American Journal of Hygiene, 53,* 262–282.

Lilienfeld, A. M., & Pasamanick, B. (1954). Association of maternal and fetal factors with the development of epilepsy: I. Abnormalities in the prenatal and paranatal periods. *Journal of the American Medical Association, 155,* 719–734.

McNulty, B., Smith, D., & Soper, E. (1984). *Effectiveness of early special education for handicapped children.* Denver: Colorado Department of Education.

Oelwein, P. L., Fewell, R. R., & Pruess, J. B. (1985). The efficacy of intervention at outreach sites of the program for children with Down syndrome and other developmental delays. *Topics in Early Childhood Special Education, 5,* 78–87.

Olds, D. L., Henderson, C. R., Jr., Tatelbaum, R., & Chamberlain, R. (1986). Improving the delivery of prenatal care and outcomes of pregnancy: A randomized trial of nurse home visitation. *Pediatrics, 77,* 16–28.

Olds, D. L., Henderson, C. R., Jr., Tatelbaum, R., & Chamberlain, R. (1988). Improving the life-course development of socially disadvantaged mothers: A randomized trial of nurse home visitation. *American Journal of Public Health, 78,* 1436–1445.

Olds, D. L., & Kitzman, H. (1990). Can home visitation improve the health of women and children at environmental risk? *Pediatrics, 68,* 108–115.

Peterson, N. (1987). *Early intervention for handicapped and at-risk children: An introduction to early childhood–special education.* Denver: Love.

Provence, S., & Lipton, R. C. (1962). *Infants in institutions.* New York: International Universities Press.

Ramey, C., Bryant, D., Sparling, J., & Wasik, B. (1985). Project CARE: A comparison of two early intervention strategies to prevent retarded development. *Topics in Early Childhood Special Education, 5,* 12–25.

Ramey, C., & Campbell, F. (1984). Preventive education for high-risk children: Cognitive consequences of the Carolina Abecedarian Project. *American Journal of Mental Deficiency, 88,* 515–523.

Reaves, J., & Burns, J. (1982, November). *An analysis of the impact of the handicapped children's early education program.* Washington, DC: Littlejohn (Roy) Associates. (ERIC Document Reproduction Service No. ED 224277)

Sameroff, A. J., & Chandler, M. (1975). Reproductive risk and the continuum of caretaking casualty. In F. D. Horowitz (Ed.), *Review of child development research* (Vol. 4, pp. 187–244). Chicago: University of Chicago Press.

Schweinhart, L. J., & Weikart, D. P. (1980). *Young children grow up: The effects of the Perry Preschool Program on youths through age 15.* Monograph No. 3. Ypsilanti, MI: High/Scope Educational Research Foundation.

Shore, R. (1997). *Rethinking the brain: New insights into early development.* New York: Families and Work Institute.

Skeels, H. M., & Dye, H. B. (1939). A study of the effects of differential stimulation on mentally retarded children. *Proceedings of the American Association of Mental Deficiency, 44,* 114–136.

Spitz, R. A. (1945). Hospitalism: An inquiry into the genesis of psychiatric conditions in early childhood. *Psychoanalytic Study of the Child, 1,* 53–74.

Stock, J. R., Wnek, L. L., Newborg, J. A., Schenck, E. A., Gabel, J. R., Spurgeon, M. S., & Ray, H. W. (1976). *Evaluation of the handicapped children's early education program.* Columbus, OH: Battelle Memorial Institute.

Upshur, C. C. (1990). Early intervention as preventive intervention. In S. J. Meisels & J. P. Shonkoff (Eds.), *Handbook of early childhood intervention* (pp. 633–650). New York: Cambridge University Press.

Vincent, L. J., Salisbury, C. L., Strain, P., McCormick, C., & Tessier, A. (1990). A behavioral-ecological approach to early intervention: Focus on cultural diversity. In S. J. Meisels & J. P. Shonkoff (Eds.), *Handbook of early childhood intervention* (pp. 173–195). New York: Cambridge University Press.

Watson, J. B. (1928). *Psychological care of the infant and child.* New York: Norton.

Weiss, H., & Halpern, R. (1991, December). *Community-based family support and education programs: Something old or something new?* New York: Columbia University, National Center for Children in Poverty. (ERIC Document Reproduction Service No. ED 341743)

Werner, E. E. (1987, July 15). *Vulnerability and resiliency: A longitudinal study of Asian-Americans from birth to age 30.* Address at the Ninth Biennial Meeting of the International Society for the Study of Behavioral Development, Tokyo.

Werner, E. E. (1989). High-risk children in young adulthood: A longitudinal study from birth to 32 years. *American Journal of Orthopsychiatry, 59,* 72–81.

Werner, E. E. (1990). Protective factors and individual resilience. In S. J. Meisels & J. P. Shonkoff (Eds.), *Handbook of early childhood intervention* (pp. 97–116). New York: Cambridge University Press.

Werner, E. E., Bierman, J. S., & French, F. E. (1971). *The children of Kauai: A longitudinal study from the prenatal period to age ten.* Honolulu: University of Hawaii Press.

Werner, E. E., & Smith, R. S. (1977). *Kauai's children come of age.* Honolulu: University of Hawaii Press.

Werner, E. E., & Smith, R. S. (1982). *Vulnerable but invincible: A longitudinal study of resilient children and youth.* New York: McGraw-Hill.

Wohlwill, J. (1973). The concept of experience: S or R? *Human Development, 16,* 90–107.

Zigler, E., & Valentine, J. (Eds.). (1979). *Project Head Start: A legacy of the War on Poverty.* New York: Free Press.

TWO

A Solid Foundation:
Knowledge Bases
to Inform Practice

I have worked for 12 years with school-age kids with special needs, and I feel pretty confident about what I have to offer to parents and children. Now I'm moving into a new position with the early intervention program in our school district, and I think I'm in over my head! I see now that working with babies and their families is a whole different ball game! Most of my coworkers are in the same boat. I guess we'll sink or float together.

—DONNA, Special Educator

Donna's situation and feelings are not unusual. Many professionals involved in the early intervention enterprise are challenged in new ways, stretched to move beyond their own professional comfort level. School psychologists and special educators often find that their practices with school-age children, or even older preschoolers, do not translate well to the birth-to-3-year-old population. Nurses used to a well-defined focus on health care sometimes find themselves challenged to function like psychologists or social workers as they grapple with the broader issues that impinge on the young child's physical development and health. Social workers may feel at a loss to understand infant development as it interfaces with the parents' own developmental issues and life circumstances. Serving infants and toddlers does not lend itself to easy compartmentalization of issues (i.e., this is a health issue; that is a psychological issue; this is an educational issue). Thus, regardless of their specific discipline or professional identity, early interventionists need a common starting point for designing interventions that reflect the integration of all domains of the child's development and the complex social contexts in which that development unfolds.

Unfortunately, given that intervention with infants and toddlers is still a relatively new, evolving field, there are few simple and definitive answers as to where to begin. In Chapter 1 we discussed the history of early intervention, tracing the theory and research that provided the impetus for the current trend to intervene at the earliest possible point in the child's development. We also identified some broad trends in early intervention practice. But you may wonder, "Where can professionals in practice turn for specific ideas about how to intervene?"

Many of us naturally turn to experienced colleagues for assistance and ideas. The experience of others is an excellent resource, yet the field of early intervention is so new in many localities that practitioners often have no one to whom to turn. As we heard from Donna at the beginning of this chapter, many early interventionists are grappling with the same questions and concerns. Even if we all had someone to consult, following common practice can be misleading unless the practice is backed by documented results. Most of us can remember times when we carried out or recommended a particular practice only to find out later that the effectiveness of the practice did not hold up to research or evaluation. It's important, therefore, to look at not only what is "tried," but also what is "true."

There are three general bodies of knowledge to which we can turn for information to guide our practice: (1) prevention and intervention research that evaluates the effectiveness of specific programs and strategies; (2) clinical evidence of effective intervention; and (3) basic developmental research that attempts to identify specific factors that account for different developmental outcomes (i.e., what characteristics of the child, the family, or the larger social environment are associated with good or poor adaptation). In this chapter, we briefly discuss these bodies of knowledge, looking at what they can and cannot tell us about how to intervene, and we indicate resources to which readers may turn to stay abreast of new information as it becomes available. Rather than providing a comprehensive literature review, we present a "state-of-the-knowledge" summary that lays the foundation for the intervention themes and strategies presented in subsequent chapters. For a more thorough review and analysis of specific studies relevant to early intervention, readers are referred to the *Handbook of Early Childhood Intervention* (Meisels & Shonkoff, 1990), and Part V of the *Handbook of Infant Mental Health*, Second Edition (Zeanah, in press), which are described in the annotated list of resources at the end of this volume.

INTERVENTION EFFECTIVENESS RESEARCH:
HOW CAN WE USE IT?

One important source of information about how to intervene is the body of research that discusses the effectiveness of specific programs or approaches to early intervention and prevention. As noted in Chapter 1, many intervention studies have been conducted during the past 25 years. Although as a group they provide general support for the importance of early intervention, an examination of those studies yields more information about the enormous challenges involved in doing such research than about how to proceed in early intervention practice.

Findings of studies generally are modest, mixed, and sometimes contradictory. Limitations in the way most studies were conducted make it difficult to ascertain (1) what, if anything, was influenced by intervention; (2) how meaningful and lasting those effects were; and (3) whether positive outcomes (if and when they occur) can be accounted for by the intervention or result from something apart from the intervention (e.g., preexisting characteristics of the child or other family members, natural support networks, events beyond the control of the intervening agency). These separate aspects of a child's life may interact in complex ways with the intervention process. Because of these different factors, some interventions may be more or less effective with certain children or families than with others. A specific intervention may work well under certain conditions but not others. It is a costly and complicated process to sort out the role of intervention within the myriad of variables that influence a child's development.

Practitioners are often uncomfortable with interpreting research, but a critical eye is important as you search the intervention research literature for ideas for practice. An understanding of a few important methodological issues will help you determine how much a particular study really can tell you about effective ways to intervene. When reviewing research, it pays to be a critic! Here are some simple questions you can ask as you look through a research study in search of ideas.

What Were the Measurable Outcomes and How Were They Measured?

One of the first considerations for researchers planning an intervention study is defining the expected—or hoped-for—outcomes. *Measures of results must be carefully selected to match the goals of the intervention program.* As discussed in Chapter 1, the first generation of early intervention studies focused primarily on cognitive outcomes, specifically improvement in IQ scores and/or later school achievement. For the birth-to-3 population, interventions usually were aimed at enhancing children's sensorimotor development through home visits, in which a home visitor taught parents ways to "stimulate" their children. For these early studies, researchers almost always chose IQ tests as a means to measure success of intervention. Among studies that targeted disadvantaged children, modest advantages (i.e., differences of 6–7 IQ points) were reported for intervention subjects as compared to control subjects who did not receive the intervention (Farran, 1990). However, over time those differences disappeared as control subjects caught up. For programs begun in infancy, IQ differences were greatest (approximately 1 standard deviation) at age 3, but diminished to ½ of a standard deviation by age 4 as the performance of control subjects improved. If the goal of intervention in these studies was to promote cognitive improvement, then results could be interpreted as showing success of the intervention or not, depending on whether short- or long-term gains (or both) are considered important.

But as some of the earlier intervention experiments revealed, effects of intervention may not be apparent immediately and/or may manifest in surprising, indirect ways. Such was the case, for example, with Head Start. Initial evaluations revealed only a minimal and short-lived impact on the intellectual and school performance of Head Start participants (Cicirelli, 1969). However, in independent long-term follow-up studies that focused on attitudes and behavior, as well as academic performance, Head Start participants were doing significantly better than other low-income children who did not participate in Head Start. They were more likely to remain in school, were less likely to be held back or placed in remedial classes, and had fewer social difficulties (Lazar & Darlington, 1982; Schweinhart, Berrueta-Clement, Barnett, Epstein, & Weikart, 1985; Schweinhart & Weikart, 1980). These findings highlight the importance of long-term follow-up studies with comprehensive, far-reaching measures.

Researchers are challenged to consider the various ways that intervention might affect children and families—including possible *negative effects*—and to design studies that cover those possibilities. We typically assume that early intervention has only positive or, at the worst, neutral results, but occasionally we may be surprised. For example, researchers from both the Carolina Abecedarian Project (Haskins, 1985) and the Syracuse Project (Honig, Lally, & Mathieson, 1982) reported that children who attended their preschools showed higher rates of aggression in the early elementary years when compared to children in a control group receiving another preschool intervention. It is likely that there have been other potentially negative results of intervention, especially with some of the more intrusive, less "family-friendly" interventions, that have not been identified because researchers weren't looking for them.

Of particular relevance to this book is the later generation of interventions that set out to influence a broad range of variables associated with the healthy, competent development of young children. As noted in Chapter 1, these broad-based interventions build on the recommendations of early intervention leaders who argued persuasively in the 1970s and 1980s that the way to effect meaningful change in the lives of children was to implement comprehensive, integrative programs that enhance the abilities of the family and community to provide ongoing support and encouragement to children. Reflecting the comprehensiveness of the interventions themselves, these studies use measures designed to tap a broad array of outcomes such as parental attitudes and beliefs, knowledge of child development, social support, coping strategies, parental mood, parent–child interactions, general family functioning, as well as the child's performance across various domains of development (see reviews by Dunst, Snyder, & Mankinen, 1989; Heinicke, Beckwith, & Thompson, 1988; Meisels, Dichtelmiller, & Liaw, 1993).

Although most analysts view these broader studies as a significant step forward in the field of early intervention, their comprehensiveness can be viewed as both an asset (from a service point of view) and a liability (from a research point of view). From a researcher's perspective, such comprehensiveness of service makes it virtually impossible to determine specifically which intervention strategies are responsible for outcomes. The most that usually can be said from such studies is that comprehensive interventions are related to positive outcomes for children and families. If a fiscal crisis or budget problems forced cuts in such a comprehensive program, it would be difficult to decide which aspect of the program to cut while maintaining positive outcomes.

It is also important to look closely at the tests, questionnaires, surveys, or other measurement devices that were used to evaluate the intervention. *Results of studies are only as good as the measures used to assess outcomes.* Assessing the development of infants and toddlers is fraught with problems. Young children's behavior is highly variable and sensitive to changes in time and setting. Besides, babies rarely perform on demand! Measures of infant and toddler behavior often lack reliability (i.e., they are not stable over time or across circumstances) and have little or no predictive validity (i.e., they do not accurately predict outcomes). Good studies always will discuss the reliability and validity of the measures used. Acceptable levels of reliability and validity range from .80 to .90 in studies with older children whose behavior is more stable. With infants and toddlers, lower levels may be acceptable; but if a study does not report them at all, the reader has no way to judge if measures used were adequate. Thus it is often difficult to draw firm conclusions from assessment results.

Even when assessing families or the broader social environment, it is challenging to find or create measures that accurately evaluate outcomes. Observational measures often are viewed as the most valid and reliable, but they are sometimes considered an invasion of family privacy and/or may be compromised by the subjects' awareness of being observed. A popular alternative, self-report measures, may elicit responses that are less than accurate, reflecting either the respondent's desire to answer in the most socially acceptable way or, in some cases, to appear more troubled as a way of crying for help.

In summary, as consumers of research findings, one of our first steps should be to look critically at how outcomes were measured and reported. Gone are the days when a simple pre–post assessment using an IQ test could be considered of much value in determining whether an intervention program is meeting its goals. Appropriate evaluation of outcomes requires a multidimensional approach using reliable and valid measures and gathering data from various sources in diverse ways.

Better Outcomes Compared to What?

One of the most critical questions when considering outcomes for intervention participants is "Compared to what?" That is, to what or whom are outcomes compared in order to determine whether participants are doing better than they would have without intervention? Some studies use a pre- and posttest design, examining changes over time for children or families participating in intervention. However, such designs do not tell us whether the observed change was due to intervention or might have occurred regardless of intervention. Particularly with infants and toddlers, development is so rapid and often uneven that a pre–post design is of little value. Even when measures assess aspects of family functioning or parental knowledge or attitudes, there is no way of knowing to what extent changes would have occurred without intervention. It is reasonable to assume that knowledge, attitudes, and family functioning change naturally with the experience of parenting.

Some intervention studies, particularly with young children with disabilities, have used *rate* of development as a pre–post measure, rather than a static assessment of performance (Bagnato & Neisworth, 1980; Wolery, 1983). That is, rather than merely looking at a child's developmental age prior to and following intervention and comparing the two, researchers may choose to look at the child's rate of development before receiving intervention and again after receiving intervention to see if the rate remained the same, increased, or decreased. But, as Farran (1990) notes, achieving a valid measure of rate of development is also highly problematic.

An alternative to pre- and posttest designs is the use of comparison groups, the most sound methodology for intervention research if the intervention and comparison groups can be assumed to be equivalent. To ensure that groups are as similar as possible, the optimal approach, from a scientific perspective, is random assignment of subjects to treatment or control group. From a service perspective, however, random assignment poses an ethical dilemma regarding denial of service to children of families who might need, or at least benefit from, the intervention. To identify a group of 20 children, for example, who appear to need intervention and to provide it to only 10 of them is at best uncomfortable and at worst illegal (in cases where the law requires us to serve all eligible children). Random assignment has been used in a number of recent studies of families who are "at risk" for poor outcomes, but have not been identified or diagnosed as having a specific problem. But in cases in which a child has an identifiable disability or when the family is asking for, or is obviously in need of, intervention, assignment to a control group usually is not acceptable or appropriate.

There are several alternatives to random assignment of subjects. Probably the next best option from a research perspective is a matched comparison group, that is, subjects who are just like the intervention participants on certain variables that might be expected to influence outcomes (e.g., SES, ethnicity, age, education, family composition, severity of disability). For example, Lovaas (1987) studied the effects of early intervention with autistic children by comparing the children who received "intensive treatment" with another group of autistic children matched on SES, family education, and other variables but receiving only minimal contact with the treatment program because they lived too far from the treatment center to receive intensive treatment. Sandow and her colleagues (Sandow & Clarke, 1978; Sandow, Clarke, Cox, & Stewart, 1981) compared outcomes for children receiving home-based services every week to a matched group of children receiving the same services every 2 months. (It's interesting to note that the children receiving services weekly made more progress during the first year of the program; however, during the second year, the bimonthly group made greater progress. The authors of this research interpreted this finding as perhaps showing that less frequent visits encouraged parents to work more independently at providing services themselves. This is another good example of the need to look at long-term, broad-based outcome measures rather than simply assuming that more is always better.)

Another option for researchers is a time-lag design in which a comparison group is recruited from the same population to be served, but is enrolled either before or after intervention participants are recruited. For example, a large Twin Cities hospital recently recruited 50 high-risk obstetric patients for a home visit intervention program. The staff then recruited the next 50 patients who had similar scores on a risk checklist to be followed as a comparison group for purposes of evaluating the impact of the home visit intervention program. Such a design assumes that the time difference between the two cohorts will not significantly influence the outcomes. However, research designs that incorporate a much greater time-lag than this may be questionable. Regardless of the type of comparison group that is used, it is important for the researchers to document the experiences of that group as carefully as possible. With the recent proliferation of programs for families and young children, control or comparison group subjects may end up inadvertently receiving other services that are similar to those provided in the intervention program that is being evaluated. Needless to say, this would make it difficult to demonstrate the impact of the intervention being studied.

The alternatives to random assignment that we describe here make it more difficult to assume equivalence of control and intervention subjects. However, they sometimes are more acceptable designs from a service perspective. Withholding service from a child or family for the sake of having a pure control group poses a serious ethical dilemma. Intervention researchers walk a fine line as they strive for an acceptable balance of the interests of science and practice. The popular 1993 motion picture *Lorenzo's Oil* reflects the perspective of many parents on the delicate balance between scientific rigor and a child's need for immediate intervention. This film tells the story of a family's desperate struggle to get treatment for their son's life-threatening degenerative nerve disorder while researchers urge them to wait until scientific studies are definitive. Although an extreme case, Lorenzo's story dramatically illustrates the dilemmas we confront as we try to understand what works and for whom.

What Actually Happened?

Another critical consideration in intervention research is documenting what actually happens in the program being studied. In the intervention research literature, interventions often are not described well, if at all. (That certainly makes it difficult to draw implications for practice! If we don't know how they did it, how can we duplicate it?) In other cases, the program may be described thoroughly, but there may be a significant difference between how an intervention is described on paper and how it actually is implemented. The "integrity" of a program (i.e., how well the program actually does what it intends to do) will vary as a function of many factors, including training and supervision of staff, different levels of commitment among staff, personality characteristics of the interveners, different levels of participation and investment on the part of the families enrolled in the program, and different needs and strengths of participants, which in turn influence what specific intervention strategies are carried out.

Another critical variable influencing program integrity is the intervener's belief in the usefulness and importance of the program. This has been cited as a major underlying factor in the so-called "generation effect," whereby a program loses its effectiveness when it is implemented by new people in a new setting following an effective initial implementation. Apparently, as the newness, excitement, and passion wear off—and as new interveners learn the program but probably do not internalize its philosophy in the way its founders have—the program may become diluted in various ways, significantly diminishing its effectiveness.

INTERVENTION RESEARCH: WHAT HAS IT TOLD US?

Despite the methodological problems discussed in the previous section, there are some general conclusions that can be drawn from the current body of research on early intervention. Drawing on several comprehensive review articles over the last decade (e.g., Barnett, 1995; Dunst et al., 1989; Meisels et al., 1993), we have selected the points that are likely to be most relevant to readers of this book. We highlight here common themes and general recommendations, both for practice and research.

General Conclusions

- Most children who receive early intervention services do make progress. How much of that progress is actually due to the early intervention services versus other factors is still a question.
- There is more evidence attesting to the effectiveness of intervention with children who are environmentally at risk than those who are biologically at risk. It is important to note that studies of biologically at-risk children usually have focused only on child outcomes, whereas research with environmentally at-risk children has used both intervention approaches and outcome measures that are more broad based.
- Thus far, findings suggest that intervention leads to greater progress for children who are higher functioning at the time of entry into the program. And, for children with disabilities, the more severe the impairment, the less progress is evident in response to intervention.
- Support for the family is a critical component of intervention. In

fact, support provided by interveners, as well as support from other out-side sources, is important to effective family functioning and, to a lesser degree, child functioning.

• The effectiveness of intervention depends on duration and age of entry into the program. This conclusion, emphasized by Dunst and his colleagues (Dunst et al., 1989), is supported also by findings based on an analysis of 20 early intervention studies that specifically set out to change some aspect of family functioning (Heinicke et al., 1988). Those authors reported that effective programs were those that began service near the time of the child's birth and continued for at least 3 months (with a minimum of 11 contacts). Time was allowed for interveners to build rapport and a sense of trust with the families served, often begin-ning by providing help with simple, concrete tasks. Openness to dealing with more personal, emotional issues usually followed, leading to incre-mental changes in the way the families communicated and coped with those issues.

• More intensive interventions are more effective than less intensive interventions, in general. At least one study raises an interesting ques-tion, however, as to how long such intensive intervention continues to be effective and/or advisable. In a 3-year intervention with parents of young children with disabilities, Sandow and colleagues (1981) found that after the first year, the more intensive intervention (2 to 3 hours per week) imparted no advantage over a less intense program (a 2- to 3-hour visit every other month). Many experts now recommend intensive services initially, with intensity later adjusted to suit the needs of the family. That, in fact, is a standard for programs seeking to be credentialed by Healthy Families America, with at least weekly services required for the first 9 months (National Committee to Prevent Child Abuse, 1997).

• Even in cases where intervention is judged to be effective, its impact is modest (i.e., accounting for about 10% of the variance in out-comes). Furthermore, because there is likely to be a publication bias, with studies demonstrating no effect being less likely to be published, it is reasonable to assume that what is in the published literature might overestimate the effectiveness of early intervention. Thus it is important to maintain realistically modest expectations in regard to the potential impact of early intervention.

Recommendations for Practice and Research

• Intervention programs should be designed within clearly defined conceptual and theoretical frameworks and should be based on the latest available knowledge about effective intervention. Consequently, even if reviewing research is not among your favorite activities, you owe it to your clients to "bite the bullet" and make it a goal to keep up on research findings.

• Interventions should be broad based, recognizing the multiple contexts in which families and children function. If your intervention focuses on working with a family in isolation (or, worse, a child in isolation), there is much you can do to increase your effectiveness.

• Interventions should be driven by the family's needs to the greatest extent possible, rather than by preplanned activities or curricula. Particularly when you are in new and unfamiliar territory, it is comforting to have a curriculum to fall back on. Yet your preplanned activities may be meaningless in the context of a particular family's needs. Flexibility and responsivity are key.

• Early interventionists must conduct evaluations of their programs, asking not only if a program works, but for whom and under what conditions. They must also try to identify what specific variables can be altered through intervention. Evaluation must adhere to the highest possible scientific standards and should be designed and used to provide feedback on an ongoing basis in order to refine and improve the quality of service.

• To compensate for small sample sizes, programs should consider pooling data to evaluate their effectiveness. This would demand, however, that programs have comparable goals, strategies, and outcome measures. Find out who else is doing what you are doing, and work together.

As researchers become more sophisticated, both in the development of intervention strategies and the design of methodologically rigorous studies of effectiveness, the knowledge available to professionals in practice will continue to grow at a dramatic rate. To stay abreast of developments in this field you may turn to scientific journals such as the *Journal of Early Intervention* (formerly the *Journal of the Division for Early Childhood,* listed under The Council for Exceptional Children), *Early Education and Development, Topics in Early Childhood Special Education,* and *Early Childhood Research Quarterly.* A few publications also provide thoughtful summaries of early intervention research, presented in a style that is easily understood by practitioners with less experience in statistics and interpretation of research findings. These include *Young Children* and *Infants and Young Children.* Information about these publications is provided in the annotated bibliography in the Appendix of this book. You will need to use a critical eye as you study the intervention research for implications for practice, keeping in mind the methodological considerations discussed in this chapter.

Clinical Evidence of Effectiveness of Intervention

A second body of knowledge that can inform practice is clinical evidence of effective intervention with individual children or families. Instead of drawing conclusions from studies of large groups, this body of knowledge is founded on an accumulation of observations from case studies and small-group interventions as practitioners work with children and families. Although often considered less scientifically rigorous than large group empirical studies, clinical evidence nevertheless can lead to useful hypotheses that help to set directions for our work with families and young children. Clinical research also has an advantage of taking into account results that lie outside the typical outcomes seen when results from large groups of children or families are lumped together.

Themes and strategies that appear repeatedly among clinical reports from different practitioners warrant particular attention and consideration as possible directions for our own practice. For example, there are numerous case studies and small-group studies that show positive outcomes when interveners support and build on family strengths rather than usurping the family's role in making decisions and providing assistance to their child (see, e.g., Brinckerhoff & Vincent, 1986; Dunst, Trivette, & Deal, 1988; Weissbourd, 1993). Although many of the earliest attempts at working with families of young children were chiefly attempts to "teach" them to stimulate their children, an accumulation of clinical research has turned the tide. We now understand that a different approach is more effective and long-lasting, that is, helping families identify and/or clarify their needs, access the resources and supports that will help them meet these needs, and exercise and hone their decision-making and problem-solving skills so that they strengthen their own capabilities (Dunst, Johanson, Trivette, & Hamby, 1991). This process will be discussed in more detail in Chapter 5.

Many other useful techniques for working with infants and their parents have been identified through clinical research and will be discussed later. For example, clinical research has been the source of ideas on the use of videotapes of parent–infant interaction to help parents recognize and modify their ways of interacting with their child, techniques for developing trusting relationships between the intervener and client, and systematic procedures for helping parents understand the link between their childhood memories and current parental behavior (see, e.g., Erickson, Korfmacher, & Egeland, 1992; Lieberman & Pawl, 1988; McDonough, 1993).

There appears to be a trend toward publishing more clinical articles and case studies from research in progress in recent years. In research reports that summarize findings for large-group data, a great deal of information about what actually went on with specific children and families is inevitably lost. Thus these clinical reports and case studies are a welcome addition to the intervention literature. *Zero to Three* and the *Family Resource Coalition Report*, described in the annotated list of resources at the end of this book, are two excellent sources of clinical information about interventions with young children and their families.

Basic Developmental Research: Implications for Intervention

The third, and very important, body of knowledge derives from studies that follow the development of young children and attempt to identify factors that are associated with good and poor developmental outcomes. To make sense of this body of research, it may be helpful to begin by defining some basic terms that are commonly used in the literature. The first term is *competence*, which refers to the effectiveness of the child's adaptation to the day-to-day ups and downs of life. This is the outward manifestation of "good developmental outcomes." Sometimes competence is equated with intellectual prowess or a set of skills within a specific domain of development. However, we are speaking here of something much broader that to a certain extent is independent of, and actually may transcend, intellectual ability. A person may be very bright, but not particularly competent in daily living. Or a person may face special intellectual challenges, but be quite competent. For example, a young boy we know has Down syndrome and tests at about 60 on a standardized IQ test. However, we would describe him as very competent. When tasks are within his ability, he does them independently, with initiative, enthusiasm, and persistence. When he reaches the limits of his own ability and internal resources, he willingly seeks and accepts help from others. And he seeks and gives comfort, warmth, and joy through his interactions with others.

A second term used to summarize developmental outcomes as they affect a child's emotional adjustment is *well-being*. This term refers to how the child feels and thinks about him- or herself and the joy and satisfaction that the child experiences in regard to his or her relationships and accomplishments. Competence and well-being may be quite independent of each other. On the one hand, a person who is outwardly competent in handling life's challenges may or may not experience a personal sense of well-being. On the other hand, a person may feel fine about him- or herself, but not demonstrate competence in negotiating life's daily challenges.

Two other crucial terms in the developmental literature are *risk factors* and *protective mechanisms*. Risk factors are characteristics of the child, the family, or the broader environment that decrease the likelihood that the child will be competent and have a sense of well-being. Protective mechanisms are factors in the child, family, or broader environment that provide a buffer against the impact of risk factors and increase the likelihood that the child will be competent and have a sense of well-being.

The developmental research that is especially relevant to early intervention is that which follows children *prospectively*. The term *prospective research* can be contrasted with *retrospective research*. In retrospective research, investigators look backward in time at child's characteristics, parental characteristics, family functioning, major life events, and aspects of the broader environment that might have influenced a child's current developmental status. For example, much of the early research on the causes of child abuse, using retrospective methods, implied that abused children came from families experiencing severe stress and that parents who abuse their children had been victims of child abuse themselves. What that research didn't tell us was why some parents experiencing severe stress or having experienced abuse as children do *not* abuse their children (e.g., Egeland & Sroufe, 1981; Egeland, Jacobvitz, & Sroufe, 1988). In prospective research, because children are followed over time, it is easier to determine why some experience certain outcomes and some do not. It allows us to look at the complexities of development (e.g., a parent who was abused as a child is likely to abuse his or her children if these factors are present, but not if those other mechanisms are operating) rather than assuming a linear model (e.g., a parent who was abused as a child abuses his or her children).

As noted in Chapter 1, several important studies have been conducted in recent years and have fueled the movement toward intervening in the earliest months of life. Such research addresses the important questions of what are the factors that increase the likelihood that a child will have problems (i.e., risk factors) and what are the factors that increase the likelihood that the child will do well (i.e., protective mechanisms). The answers to those questions can be very helpful in guiding early intervention efforts. In fact, one way to define the goal of early intervention is to tip the balance in favor of protective mechanisms, that is, to eliminate or diminish risk factors where it is possible, and to create or enhance protective mechanisms that will serve as a buffer against the risk factors that remain. (Keep in mind that "risk" is a relative concept; we all have risk factors and protective mechanisms operating in our lives, as do the children and families with whom we work.)

So, what specifically does developmental research tell us about the risk factors and protective mechanisms that are most critical to the development of competence and well-being? And most importantly, which are the factors that we realistically might hope to change through early intervention? Several factors have emerged repeatedly in studies of different populations and thus deserve careful consideration in the planning of intervention programs.

RELATIONSHIPS WITH CARING, TRUSTWORTHY ADULTS

One of the most critical variables identified in most studies of child development is the child's relationship with a supportive adult. The absence of close, supportive relationships with adult caregivers appears to put children at risk for varied and multiple problems, particularly in the domain of social–emotional development. On the other hand, experience with a caring, trusted adult facilitates the child's optimal development. Such a relationship can serve as a powerful protective mechanism. Even in the face of abuse or other trauma or hardship, the presence of a supportive adult may be the factor that allows the child to bounce back and develop competence and well-being (Blum & Rinehart, 1997; Egeland & Sroufe, 1981; Garmezy, 1987; Werner, 1990;). The key adult who makes a difference for a child may be a member of the child's immediate or extended family, an adult friend of the family, a teacher, a pastor, or a youth leader.

Of course, in the early months or years of a child's life—the time with which we are most concerned in this book—the circle of adults in the child's life is usually relatively small. Much of the infant's or toddler's time is spent with parents or other family members. A rapidly growing body of research points to those earliest relationships as a strong and lasting influence on the child's ongoing development. In particular, research guided by attachment theory has provided strong evidence of the importance of the infant–caregiver relationship in laying a secure foundation on which later development builds.

For example, several studies have documented the relationship between quality of attachment in infancy and later social behavior and school achievement (e.g., Erickson, Sroufe, & Egeland, 1985; Lewis, Feiring, McGuffog, & Jaskir, 1984; Sroufe & Jacobvitz, 1989; Urban, Carlson, Egeland, & Sroufe, 1991). It appears that this early primary attachment helps to determine the child's sense of self, expectations of others, and patterns of behavior in later relationships. (As Zeanah [1997] notes, even if a secure relationship did not predict later behavior, it is a central part of the infant's quality of life in the here and now.) Thus developmental research suggests that one logical goal of early intervention would be to support and promote the development of secure attachment between the infant and his or her caregivers.

Developmental research also offers some guidance as to how that might be accomplished, that is, by what pathway a secure attachment develops. Among the factors that influence quality of attachment, a particularly critical variable appears to be *the sensitivity of the caregiver to the infant's cues and signals* (Ainsworth, Blehar, Waters, & Wall, 1978; DeWolff & van IJzendoorn, 1997; Egeland & Farber, 1984). Parental sensitivity has been related to other positive outcomes as well, including a higher level of mastery motivation (Yarrow, Rubenstein, & Pederson, 1975) and higher intellectual functioning at subsequent ages (Beckwith, Cohen, Kopp, Parmelee, & Marcy, 1976; Bradley & Caldwell, 1984; Coates & Lewis, 1984). Most recently, neuroscientists have begun to document the effects of sensitive care on the physiological development of the brain, which in turn affects learning and behavior across the lifespan (Shore, 1997).

The challenge to early interventionists then is to determine how to support parents in (1) learning to read their infants' cues and (2) maintaining the emotional energy necessary to sustain an adequately sensitive level of responding. This demands an ecological or systems approach that takes into account the many factors that can influence, and be influenced by, parental sensitivity (Cowan, 1997). (In Chapter 3, we discuss attachment in some detail, describing different patterns of attachment, discussing parental sensitivity and other factors associated with secure and insecure patterns, and suggesting intervention strategies for enhancing parental sensitivity and promoting the development of secure attachment.)

OTHER PARENTAL BEHAVIORS THAT FACILITATE OPTIMAL DEVELOPMENT

While parental sensitivity emerges as one of the most—if not *the* most—important aspects of the caregiver–child relationship for promoting good development, research points as well to other important behaviors during the infant and toddler period. *Talking to babies*, even long before they comprehend or can speak words, is important to good development. Not surprisingly, talking (or singing or reading) to babies long has been known to be a factor in promoting language development (Clarke-Stewart, 1973). The parent's voice also serves an important function as a source of comfort to the baby (Nugent, 1985).

Yet some parents do not recognize the importance of talking to their infants. Several studies have shown that teen parents talk less to their babies than older parents (e.g., Epstein, 1980; Osofsky & Osofsky, 1970), a factor that may account at least in part for the poorer achievement and language skills of children born to teen parents. And more recently, Hart and Risley (1995) have provided dramatic evidence attesting to the long-term consequences for young children growing up with parents who seldom talk to them. (In our own work we have heard parents ask, "Why talk to her when she can't understand anyway?") Also important is reading to babies, a way of introducing them to the world of learning through books, sharing with them the joy of words and pictures. This again is something parents may not pursue because the baby does not "understand," or because the parents themselves may lack reading skills or interest.

As babies become mobile and able to explore and manipulate objects in their environment, the role of the parent in *facilitating and encouraging that exploration* becomes very important to the child's development. Studies have shown a relationship between school success and opportunities during infancy to play with a variety of materials in a relatively unrestricted physical environment (Bradley & Caldwell, 1984). A child's opportunity to explore may be limited by such factors as overcrowded and unsafe physical environments, restrictive parental attitudes, or a child's physical or sensory disabilities. Thus, one role of early intervention may be to work with the family to overcome those obstacles so that the child can explore freely.

Children not only need a chance to explore the environment, but to master it (Lyons-Ruth & Zeanah, 1993; MacTurk, McCarthy, Vietze, & Yarrow, 1987; MacTurk, Vietze, McCarthy, McQuiston, & Yarrow, 1985). The task for parents is to *create situations where a goal is attainable* with some effort on the part of the child. Thus a task for early intervention may be to help parents understand the importance of mastery experiences and discover ways to enable the child to have those experiences, regardless of any special challenges imposed by biology or environment. The parental role is to provide just enough help and support to allow the child to succeed and feel that he or she is responsible for the accomplishment (Lyons-Ruth & Zeanah, 1993; Matas, Arend, & Sroufe, 1978).

As the baby moves into the toddler phase, when autonomy or independence is the central developmental issue (Erikson, 1963), it is increasingly important that parents strike a balance between too much help and too little. Parent–child difficulties around autonomy issues at age 2 have been associated with behavior problems at later ages (e.g., Block, 1971; Erickson, Sroufe, & Egeland, 1985; Martin, 1981). Without help and support, the toddler faces frustration and learns that he or she is incompetent and others are unavailable. With too much help, the child gets the message that others have to solve the problem because he or she is incapable. "Balance" also seems to be the key word in regard to discipline and limit setting during the toddler period. Many classic studies of parent–child relations have demonstrated the importance of setting clear, consistent limits, balanced by opportunities for choice and autonomy (Baumrind, 1967, 1971; Lytton, 1977; Schaffer & Crook, 1980).

PARENTAL KNOWLEDGE, BELIEFS, AND ATTITUDES

To a large extent, parental behavior is a function of what parents know, understand, and believe about how children develop and learn (see Sigel, 1985, for a thorough discussion of parental beliefs and child development). Several aspects of parental knowledge and beliefs emerge from developmental research as being especially important during the infant and toddler periods. First of all is a recognition of the capabilities of the newborn. Some parents have a view of the newborn as a doll, overlooking the remarkable capabilities of the infant to communicate needs and feelings. Other parents may attribute too much understanding or intentionality to a young baby, saying, for example, that a crying 3-month-old boy is "getting back" at them for leaving him with a babysitter last night. In either case, this lack of recognition of a baby's capabilities may underlie a parent's inability to see things from the infant's perspective and may, in part, account for apparent insensitivity to the baby's cues and signals.

A related issue is *knowledge of developmental sequences* and normal, expected behavior at different points in the child's development, a knowledge that helps to determine parents' expectations for their child's behavior. Unrealistic expectations (e.g., expecting a 1-year-old to sit still and listen) have been shown to be associated with abuse and with other negative outcomes for parents and children (Newberger & Cook, 1983). Perhaps even more important than simple knowledge of developmental sequences is *understanding the meaning of the child's behavior.* Parental misunderstanding can lead to negative attributions toward the child and/ or self (Egeland & Breitenbucher, 1980; Erickson et al., 1992; Newberger & Cook, 1983). For example, a mother who does not understand the meaning of an 8-month-old's separation anxiety may think that the baby is "spoiled" and/or she may feel like a "bad" mother. With a child with disabilities, understanding behavior and setting realistic expectations is much more complex and may require careful observation and experimentation to figure out the child's capabilities, needs, and feelings.

For some parents, even when they have accurate knowledge and understanding of their child's development, and have formed realistic expectations for their child's behavior, their own emotional issues make it difficult for them to put that knowledge into practice. A special subset of parental attitudes involves thoughts and feelings about their own upbringings. Recent research demonstrates the relationship between a parent's thoughts about his or her own childhood and the way that parent interacts with his or her baby (van IJzendoorn, 1995; Zeanah et al., 1993). Specifically, parents who form secure, healthy attachments with their children usually have faced the negative, painful things they experienced in their relationships with their own parents, and they recognize that the way they were parented has a powerful influence on their interactions with their own children. They have come to some level of resolution that allows them to move toward new ways of caring for their children, choosing what to repeat and not repeat from their past.

On the other hand, parents are more likely to have attachment problems, or even to maltreat their children, if they deny, dismiss, or remain preoccupied with the pain from their own past (Main, 1995; Main & Goldwyn, 1984; Main & Hesse, 1990). These findings point to the importance of going beyond simple parent education to address the deeper emotional issues that may make it difficult for a parent to put his or her knowledge to work in a relationship with the child. We discuss this in more detail in Chapter 4.

SOCIAL SUPPORT FOR THE FAMILY

Parenting is not a solitary endeavor and there is a great deal of evidence showing the importance of social support as a key factor in enabling a parent to do his or her job well (Kagan, Powell, Weissbourd, & Zigler, 1987; Powell, 1987). The relatively high incidence of problems among children of single parents is well documented. However, support goes well beyond having a spouse. Many married parents may not receive or provide adequate mutual support. Nor, of course, is a partner the only viable source of support. Young, single mothers who care well for children, promoting their optimal development, usually have good support from someone—their own parent, another relative, or a close friend. Even for two-parent families with strong, supportive marriages, the presence of a caring extended family and community makes a difference.

Support may come from formal resources as well (e.g., religious organizations, professional helpers, intervention agencies), but, as Dunst et al. (1988) caution, service providers should in no way supplant the natural support network of a family. Based on their review of research on social support, Dunst and colleagues emphasize that studies consistently show informal support (i.e., individuals and social groups that provide support as a result of daily informal contact with families) to be much more effective than formal support (i.e., professionals and agencies working toward this purpose). However, rather than discouraging those of us who work in formal agencies, this finding should encourage us to identify, understand, and work with rather than against these informal sources of support as we attempt to assist children and their families.

Social support has been shown to make a difference for mothers of premature infants (Crnic, Greenberg, Ragozin, Robinson, & Basham, 1983), adolescent mothers (Colletta, 1981), parents whose children are making the transition from the neonatal intensive care unit to home (Affleck, Tennen, Allen, & Gershman, 1986), and parents of other high-risk infants (Crnic, Greenberg, & Slough, 1986). In some cases, supportive resources are available, but parents do not use them effectively. Barriers to effective use of formal resources include lack of transportation, insufficient money, and bureaucratic obstacles such as unwieldy paperwork, unhelpful staff, and incomprehensible regulations. Parents also may be reluctant to accept, or unsure of how to ask for, help and support within the natural support network. Early intervention can and should be a source of support in and of itself; but, more importantly, it can help parents to identify supportive resources and overcome barriers to using those resources. Chapter 5 provides more information about these topics.

SUMMARY

Each of these three bodies of knowledge (intervention research, clinical evidence, and basic developmental research) has its limitations. The relatively modest findings of intervention studies lead only to broad conclusions, seldom providing specific guidance. Clinical evidence from work with individual families and children yields useful ideas for practice, but lacks the statistical power to indicate potential effectiveness with other families. Developmental research identifies critical variables that have been shown to relate to different outcomes for children and families. But that research tells us little about to what extent those variables can be changed—or, if they are changed, whether good outcomes will follow.

Nevertheless, where these three sources of knowledge converge, we can have increased confidence that we are building our interventions on a sound foundation. Throughout all three bodies of knowledge, we encounter themes related to the importance of relationships characterized by trust, sensitivity, and encouragement (both between children and caregivers and between families and interveners). We see that intervention can indeed help children and families, but that it is important to recognize and incorporate naturally occurring events and relationships in this intervention. We find that it's usually the job of early intervention not to create, but rather to support, facilitate, identify, and build on the strengths that exist in and for each child and family. And finally, we note that no one intervention works for everyone. We must be flexible and resourceful in choosing techniques for each unique situation. There are no magic tricks or quick fixes, only these basic elements that have been important to parents and children for generations.

In the remaining chapters of this book, we describe and discuss basic practices based on these major areas of converging knowledge. Although there still are many unanswered questions about when, where, and how to influence some of these critical variables, the behaviors, attitudes, and social factors we have chosen as our focus seem to be relatively accessible and amenable to change. As such, they provide a useful starting point for assessing and working with young children and their families. It will be your responsibility to evaluate the appropriateness of these themes and the effectiveness of the suggested strategies with each child and family you serve.

REFERENCES

Affleck, G., Tennen, H., Allen, D. A., & Gershman, K. (1986). Perceived social support and maternal adaptation during the transition from hospital to home care of high-risk infants. *Infant Mental Health Journal, 7*, 6–18.

Ainsworth, M. D. S., Blehar, M. C., Waters, E., & Wall, S. (1978). *Patterns of attachment: A psychological study of the Strange Situation.* Hillsdale, NJ: Erlbaum.

Bagnato, S. J., & Neisworth, T. J. (1980). The Intervention Efficiency Index: An approach to preschool accountability. *Exceptional Children, 46,* 264–269.

Barnett, W. S. (1995). Long-term effects of early childhood programs on cognitive and school outcomes. *The Future of Children: Long-Term Outcomes of Early Childhood Programs, 5,* 25–50.

Baumrind, D. (1967). Child care practices anteceding three patterns of preschool behavior. *Genetic Psychology Monographs, 75,* 43–88.

Baumrind, D. (1971). Current patterns of parental authority. *Developmental Psychology Monograph, 4*(1, Pt. 2).

Beckwith, L., Cohen, S. E., Kopp, C. B., Parmelee, A. H., & Marcy, T. G. (1976). Caregiver–infant interaction and early cognitive development in preterm infants. *Child Development, 47,* 579–587.

Block, J. (1971). *Lives through time.* Berkeley, CA: Bancroft Books.

Blum, R. W., & Rinehart, P. M. (1997). *Reducing the risk: Connections that make a difference in the lives of youth.* Minneapolis: Division of General Pediatrics and Adolescent Health, University of Minnesota.

Bradley, R. H., & Caldwell, B. M. (1984). The relation of infants' home environment to achievement test performance in first grade: A follow-up study. *Child Development, 55,* 803–809.

Brinckerhoff, J. L., & Vincent, L. J. (1986). Increasing parental decision-making at their child's individualized educational program meeting. *Journal of the Division for Early Childhood, 2,* 46–58.

Cicirelli, V. (1969). *The impact of Head Start.* Athens, OH: Westinghouse Learning Corporation.

Clarke-Stewart, K. A. (1973). Interactions between mothers and their young children. *Monographs of the Society for Research in Child Development, 38*(7–9, Serial No. 153).

Coates, D. L., & Lewis, M. (1984). Early mother–infant interaction and infant cognitive status as predictors of school performance and cognitive behavior in 6-year-olds. *Child Development, 55,* 1219–1230.

Colletta, N. (1981). Social support and the risk of maternal rejection by adolescent mothers. *Journal of Psychology, 109,* 191–197.

Cowan, P. A. (1997). Beyond meta-analysis: A plea for a family systems view of attachment. *Child Development, 68,* 601–603.

Crnic, K. A., Greenberg, M., Ragozin, A., Robinson, N., & Basham, R. (1983). Effects of stress and social support on mothers of premature and full-term infants. *Child Development, 54,* 209–217.

Crnic, K. A., Greenberg, M. T., & Slough, N. M. (1986). Early stress and social support influences on mothers' and high-risk infants' functioning in late infancy. *Infant Mental Health Journal, 7,* 19–48.

De Wolff, M. S., & van IJzendoorn, M. H. (1997). Sensitivity and attachment: A meta-analysis on parental antecedents of infant attachment. *Child Development, 68,* 571–591.

Dunst, C. J., Johanson, C., Trivette, C. M., & Hamby, D. (1991). Family-oriented early intervention policies and practices: Family-oriented or not? *Exceptional Children, 58,* 115–126.

Dunst, C. J., Snyder, S., & Mankinen, M. (1989). Efficacy of early intervention. In M. Wang, H. Walberg, & M. Reynolds (Eds.), *Handbook of special education: Research and practice III* (pp. 259–294). Oxford, England: Pergamon Press.

Dunst, C. J., Trivette, C. M., & Deal, A. G. (1988). *Enabling and empowering families: Principles and guidelines for practice.* Cambridge, MA: Brookline Books.

Egeland, B., & Breitenbucher, M. (1980). *Final report: The effects of parental knowledge and expectations on the development of child competence* (Grant No. 90-C-1259). Washington, DC: Administration for Children, Youth and Families, Office of Child Development, Department of Health, Education and Welfare.

Egeland, B., & Farber, E. A. (1984). Infant–mother attachment: Factors related to its development and changes over time. *Child Development, 55,* 753–771.

Egeland, B., Jacobvitz, D., & Sroufe, L. A. (1988). Breaking the cycle of abuse. *Child Development, 59,* 1080–1088.

Egeland, B., & Sroufe, L. A. (1981). Developmental sequelae of maltreatment in infancy. In R. Rizley & D. Cicchetti (Eds.), *New directions in child development: Developmental perspectives in child maltreatment* (pp. 77–92). San Francisco: Jossey-Bass.

Epstein, A. S. (1980). *Assessing the child development information needed by adolescent parents with very young children.* Ypsilanti, MI: High/Scope

Educational Research Foundation. (ERIC Document Reproduction Service No. ED 183 286)

Erickson, M. F., Korfmacher, J., & Egeland, B. (1992). Attachments past and present: Implications for therapeutic intervention with mother–infant dyads. *Development and Psychopathology, 4,* 495–507.

Erickson, M. F., Sroufe, L. A., & Egeland, B. (1985). The relationship between quality of attachment and behavior problems in preschool in a high-risk sample. In I. Bretherton & E. Waters (Eds.), Growing points of attachment theory and research. *Monographs of the Society for Research in Child Development, 50*(1–2, Serial No. 209), 147–166.

Erikson, E. (1963). *Childhood and society* (2nd ed.). New York: Norton.

Farran, D. C. (1990). Effects of intervention with disadvantaged and disabled children: A decade review. In S. J. Meisels & J. P. Shonkoff (Eds.), *Handbook of early childhood intervention* (pp. 501–533). New York: Cambridge University Press.

Garmezy, N. (1987). Stress, competence, and development: Continuities in the study of schizophrenic adults, children vulnerable to psychopathology, and the search for stress-resistant children. *American Journal of Orthopsychiatry, 57,* 159–174.

Hart, B., & Risley, T. (1995). *Meaningful differences in the everyday experience of young American children.* Baltimore: Brookes.

Haskins, R. (1985). Public school aggression among children with varying day-care experience. *Child Development, 56,* 689–703.

Heinicke, C. M., Beckwith, L., & Thompson, A. (1988). Early intervention in the family systems: A framework and review. *Infant Mental Health Journal, 9,* 111–141.

Honig, A., Lally, R., & Mathieson, D. (1982). Personal–social adjustment of school children after 5 years in a family enrichment program. *Child Care Quarterly, 2,* 138–146.

Kagan, S. L., Powell, D. R., Weissbourd, B., & Zigler, E. F. (1987). *America's family support programs.* New Haven: Yale University Press.

Lazar, I., & Darlington, R. (1982). Lasting effects of early education: A report from the Consortium for Longitudinal Studies. *Monographs of the Society for Research in Child Development, 47*(2–3, Serial No. 195).

Lewis, M., Feiring, C., McGuffog, C., & Jaskir, J. (1984). Predicting psychopathology in 6-year-olds from early social relations. *Child Development, 55,* 123–136.

Lieberman, A. F., & Pawl, J. H. (1988). Clinical applications of attachment theory. In J. Belsky & T. Nezworski (Eds.), *Clinical implications of attachment* (pp. 327–348). Hillsdale, NJ: Erlbaum.

Lovaas, O. I. (1987). Behavioral treatment and normal educational and intellectual functioning in young autistic children. *Journal of Consulting and Clinical Psychology, 55,* 3–9.

Lyons-Ruth, K., & Zeanah, C. H., Jr. (1993). The family context of infant mental health: I. Affective development in the primary caregiving relationship. In C. H. Zeanah, Jr. (Ed.), *Handbook of infant mental health* (pp. 14–37). New York: Guilford Press.

Lytton, H. (1977). Correlates of compliance and the rudiments of conscience in 2-year-old boys. *Canadian Journal of Behavioral Sciences, 9,* 242–251.

MacTurk, R. H., McCarthy, M. E., Vietze, P. M., & Yarrow, L. J. (1987). Sequential analysis of mastery behavior in 6- and 12-month-old infants. *Developmental Psychology, 23,* 199–203.

MacTurk, R. H., Vietze, P. M., McCarthy, M. E., McQuiston, S., & Yarrow, L. J. (1985). The organization of exploratory behavior in Down syndrome and nondelayed infants. *Child Development, 56,* 573–581.

Main, M. (1995). Recent studies in attachment: Overview, with selected implications for clinical work. In S. Goldberg, R. Muir, & J. Kerr (Eds.), *Attachment theory: Social, developmental, and clinical perspectives* (pp. 407–474). New York: Analytic Press.

Main, M., & Goldwyn, R. (1984). Predicting rejection of her infant from mother's representation of her own experience: Implications for the abused and abusing intergenerational cycle. *Child Abuse and Neglect, 8,* 203–217.

Main, M., & Hesse, E. (1990). Parents' unresolved traumatic experiences are related to infant disorganized attachment status: Is frightened and/or frightening parental behavior the linking mechanism? In M. T. Greenberg, D. Cicchetti, & E. M. Cummings (Eds.), *Attachment in the preschool years* (pp. 161–182). Chicago: University of Chicago Press.

Martin, J. A. (1981). A longitudinal study of the consequence of early mother–infant interaction: A microanalytic approach. *Monographs of the Society for Research in Child Development, 46*(3, Serial No. 190).

Matas, L., Arend, R., & Sroufe, L. A. (1978). Continuity of adaptation in the second year: The relationship between quality of attachment and later competence. *Child Development, 49,* 547–556.

McDonough, S. C. (1993). Interaction guidance: Understanding and treating early infant–caregiver relationship disturbances. In C. H. Zeanah, Jr. (Ed.), *Handbook of infant mental health* (pp. 414–426). New York: Guilford Press.

Meisels, S. J., Dichtelmiller, M., & Liaw, F. (1993). A multidimensional analysis of early childhood intervention programs. In C. H. Zeanah, Jr. (Ed.), *Handbook of infant mental health* (pp. 361–385). New York: Guilford Press.

National Committee to Prevent Child Abuse. (1997). *Healthy Families America credentialing standards.* Chicago: Author.

Newberger, C. M., & Cook, S. J. (1983). Parental awareness and child abuse: A cognitive–developmental analysis of urban and rural samples. *American Journal of Orthopsychiatry, 53,* 512–524.

Nugent, K. J. (1985). *Using the NBAS with infants and their families: Guidelines for intervention.* New York: March of Dimes.

Osofsky, H. J., & Osofsky, J. D. (1970). Adolescents as mothers: Results of a program for low-income pregnant teenagers with some emphasis upon infants' development. *American Journal of Orthopsychiatry, 40,* 825–834.

Powell, D. (Ed.). (1987). *Parent education and support programs: Consequences for children and families.* Norwood, NJ: Ablex.

Sandow, S., & Clarke, A. (1978). Home intervention with parents of severely subnormal preschool children: An interim report. *Child: Care, Health, and Development, 4,* 29–39.

Sandow, S. A., Clarke, A., Cox, M., & Stewart, F. (1981). Home intervention with parents of severely subnormal children: A final report. *Child: Care, Health, and Development, 7,* 135–144.

Schaffer, H. R., & Crook, C. K. (1980). Child compliance and maternal control techniques. *Developmental Psychology, 16,* 54–61.

Schweinhart, L., Berrueta-Clement, J., Barnett, S., Epstein, A., & Weikart, D. (1985). Effects of the Perry Preschool Program on youths through age 19: A summary. *Topics in Early Childhood Special Education, 5,* 26–35.

Schweinhart, L. J., & Weikart, D. P. (1980). *Young children grow up: The effects of the Perry Preschool Program on youths through age 15.* Monograph No. 3. Ypsilanti, MI: High/Scope Educational Research Foundation.

Shore, R. (1997). *Rethinking the brain: New insights into early development.* New York: Families and Work Institute.

Sigel, E. (1985). *Parental belief systems: The psychological consequences for children.* Hillsdale, NJ: Erlbaum.

Sroufe, L. A., & Jacobvitz, D. (1989). Diverging pathways, developmental transformations, multiple etiologies, and the problem of continuity in development. *Human Development, 32,* 196–203.

Urban, J., Carlson, E., Egeland, B., & Sroufe, L. A. (1991). Patterns of individual adaptation across childhood. *Development and Psychopathology, 4,* 445–460.

van IJzendoorn, M. H. (1995). Adult attachment representations, parental responsiveness, and infant attachment: A meta-analysis on the predictive validity of the Adult Attachment Interview. *Psychological Bulletin, 117,* 387–403.

Weissbourd, B. (1993). Family support programs. In C. H. Zeanah, Jr. (Ed.), *Handbook of infant mental health* (pp. 402–413). New York: Guilford Press.

Werner, E. E. (1990). Protective factors and individual resilience. In S. J. Meisels & J. P. Shonkoff (Eds.), *Handbook of early childhood intervention* (pp. 97–116). New York: Cambridge University Press.

Wolery, M. (1983). Proportional Change Index: An alternative for comparing child change data. *Exceptional Children, 50,* 167–170.

Yarrow, L. J., Rubenstein, J. L., & Pederson, F. A. (1975). *Infant and environment: Early cognitive and motivational development.* New York: Wiley.

Zeanah, C. H., Jr. (1997, May). *Perspectives on infant mental health: Implications for practice.* Presentation to the Minnesota Round Table on Early Childhood Education, Minneapolis, MN.

Zeanah, C. H., Jr., Benoit, D., Barton, M., Hirshberg, L., Regan, C., & Lipsitt, L. (1993). Representations of attachment in mothers and their 1-year-old infants. *Journal of the American Academy of Child and Adolescent Psychiatry, 32,* 278–286.

THREE

Identifying and Building on Parenting Strengths

When Sara grows up, I want her to be successful and happy. I want her to get along well with other people, but not to be a pushover. She'll need to know how to look out for herself and not let people take advantage of her. And she'll need to feel good about herself—you know, have good self-esteem. I have a good idea of what I want for her, but what I'm not so sure of is what I can do to see that things turn out that way. At what age will it really start to matter what I do with her? Is there anything I should be doing right now?

—LISA, mother of a 3-month-old

Lisa expresses the hopes and the questions of many new parents. In our work with parents from many walks of life, we hear the same desires and aspirations for a good life for their children. We hear parents' genuine longing to do what they can to make their dreams come true for their children. And, we hear searching questions about what really will matter—the what, how, when, where, and why of parenting. Regardless of age, SES, cultural background, or geographic location, parents seem to share similar wishes for their children and similar questions about how to fulfill those wishes.

Of course, there are no quick, easy answers to parents' questions. There are no simple instruction manuals to tell us how to create a child who is "successful and happy," as Lisa hopes her daughter will be. There are many forces at work in children's lives, and, although parental influences are powerful, they are mitigated by many other variables beyond the control of parents. Nevertheless, there *are* things that parents can do from the first day of a baby's life to promote good outcomes. And some of those things apparently matter a great deal, according to recent research.

In this chapter we focus on the overt, observable behavior of parents, specifically the dimensions of parenting behavior that have been shown to make a real difference for children's development. (Later chapters will explore the attitudes, knowledge, and feelings that underlie parenting behavior, as well as the social contexts that support or hinder parents' efforts.) We suggest what to look for when observing parents in interaction with their infants and toddlers, discuss how and why those behaviors are important to later development, and describe intervention strategies aimed at building on parenting strengths.

A FIRM FOUNDATION:
INFANT–CAREGIVER ATTACHMENT

A central issue in the first year of a child's life is the establishment of a sense of basic trust (Erikson, 1963). Through experiences with caregivers, babies are receiving important messages about the world around them: whether it is a place of love, warmth, and safety; whether it is a relatively stable, predictable place where they are cared for in a consistent way. In less optimal circumstances, a baby may experience the world as a place where others cannot be counted on; where care is unreliable, erratic, or virtually absent; or perhaps even a place where those closest to him or her are frightening or hurtful. Ideally, however, a child learns that others can be trusted, that they are there to respond and care and love in a consistent way. Along with that trust in others comes a trust in oneself, especially in one's own ability to influence and get a response from others: "When I cry, Dad comforts me. When I reach out with a smile or a laugh, Mom plays with me. I am effective in seeing that my own needs are met."

This sense of basic trust is influenced by many experiences in the young child's life, but probably is most closely tied to the child's relationship or attachment to his or her primary caregivers. These may be Mom and/or Dad, a grandparent, or whoever else spends a significant amount of time with the child *and* has a strong emotional investment in him or her. The attachment between an individual and the parents or other primary caregivers is important throughout the lifespan (in fact, in Chapter 4 we discuss how adults' thoughts and feelings about their own early attachments influence their attitudes and behavior in regard to their children). But attachment has special salience as a developmental issue during the first months of life when much of the baby's experience and learning unfolds within the context of that developing relationship.

As mentioned in Chapters 1 and 2, a growing body of literature attests to the importance of parent–infant attachment as a powerful influence on the child's development. This literature includes theoretical work, such as the prolific writing of British psychiatrist Bowlby (e.g., 1973, 1980, 1982); research that directly measures attachment and explores its role in development (much of which is discussed below); and writings that attempt to link theory and research to practice (e.g., Belsky & Nezworski, 1988; Erickson, Korfmacher, & Egeland, 1992; Greenberg, Cicchetti, & Cummings, 1990). Already attachment theory and research have had a powerful influence on early intervention with infants and their parents. And as research continues to reveal more about how attachments form and how they influence the ongoing development of the child and the family, it will be critical for those of us who serve families and young children to act on that knowledge.

How Attachments Develop

Human infants (and other primate infants as well) are predisposed to form attachments to the adults who care for them in the first few months of life. Babies come into the world with behaviors that serve to build that connection with others: sucking, clinging, grasping, and crying, to name a few. Initially, closeness with adult caregivers is essential for the physical survival of the totally dependent young baby. But infant–caregiver attachment also serves an important function in creating the context in which the baby's learning and development unfold. Although the attachment to caregiver begins to develop from the first moment of the child's life, it is not an "instant glue" kind of experience. This relationship develops gradually over weeks and months, as the baby and adult engage in repeated interactions, adapting to each other's unique ways. The attachment typically has become well established by the time the child is about 1 year of age.

It is important to note here that attachment researchers make a distinction between *attachment* and what is popularly called *bonding*. Bonding often is used to describe a relatively brief experience during the first moments or days of the baby's life, when many parents feel those first rushes of parental instinct and nurturing love. For example, we often hear people refer to parents and baby being allowed a few hours together in the mother's hospital room to "bond." Research in the 1970s suggested that such a time of bonding in the early hours or days of the infant's life was necessary to get the parent–child relationship off on the right foot (Kennell & Klaus, 1976). That research provided the impetus for hospitals to modify their care practices for mother and child to allow for greater contact between parent and newborn.

However, that research also raised the anxiety of many parents who, for one reason or another (e.g., medical complications in mother or child, hospital restrictions, or perhaps stressful events or postpartum depression that interfered with the mother's ability to engage emotionally with her infant), did not have that early bonding experience with their infant. Fortunately, subsequent research has demonstrated that although early bonding with the newborn is important, it does not make or break the parent–child relationship (e.g., Rode, Chang, Fisch, & Sroufe, 1981; Singer, Brodzinsky, Ramsay, Stein, & Waters, 1985). Whereas those early hours together can be a wonderful time for parents and baby, the short-term bonding experience is not the same as the gradual process of attachment.

Furthermore, the new infants are not sufficiently aware and comprehending to be full-partners in the so-called bonding experience. As infants mature and develop, however, they do become active, reciprocal, knowing partners in the growing attachment with caregivers. Especially when the baby achieves the cognitive milestone that Piaget (1952) called *object permanence*, (the understanding that an object exists even when it isn't in sight), the attachment becomes a two-way relationship that both partners work to maintain. In the case of attachment, the object of interest to the baby is the caregiver, and, with the attainment of the concept of object permanence, the child knows that the caregiver exists even when he or she is out of sight. So, often with a vehement cry, the baby acknowledges the absence of the caregiver and works to bring him or her back.

Thus, in the child development literature, attachment has a special meaning as a term that describes a mutual, reciprocal relationship that develops gradually over time, typically becoming well established near the end of the first year of the baby's life. Of course, that attachment continues to evolve and be manifest in different ways as the child and caregiver both develop and move into and out of different life circumstances.

Nearly all infants form attachments. Exceptions are children who have no opportunity for sustained interactions with a caregiver, for example, those in institutions or a rapid succession of foster homes. Although infant–caregiver attachments are nearly universal, they vary significantly in quality. These qualitative differences are of special interest to those of us in early intervention. Attachments can be broadly classified as *anxious* or *secure*. A secure attachment is reflected in the child's ability to use the caregiver as a secure base from which to explore the world and as a reliable source of comfort during times of distress. An anxious attachment, on the other hand, does not provide that place of comfort and stability and therefore does not serve as a safe platform from which to venture out into the world. Not surprisingly, children's ongoing development can vary notably depending on the quality of that early attachment relationship.

Assessing Quality of Attachment

Ainsworth (Ainsworth, Blehar, Waters, & Wall, 1978) was the first to develop a measure that allowed reliable assessment of the quality of infant–caregiver attachment. Based on months of observing parents and infants in naturalistic settings, across various environments and cultural contexts, she developed a 20-minute laboratory procedure designed to capture what she had observed in the day-to-day interactions of families. Called the "Strange Situation" procedure, this assessment involves bringing the child and caregiver into a small unfamiliar room and video-taping them as they interact during a series of eight brief episodes. The episodes are designed to observe the child's play and exploration in the presence and absence of the caregiver, the child's reaction to a stranger, the child's response to two brief separations from the caregiver, and, most importantly, his or her behavior when the caregiver reenters the room following the separation episodes.

Although attachments endure throughout the lifespan, this measure is designed to capture the major ways in which attachment is manifest during a specific period of development, typically when the infant is approximately 11–20 months of age. With younger infants, it would not be fair to assume that the attachment is fully established. With older toddlers or preschoolers, it would be questionable to assume that a 2-minute separation from the caregiver would be disturbing enough to tap accurately into the coping strategies of the pair.

Based on a relatively complex scheme for coding the Strange Situation videotapes, infant–caregiver pairs are classified into one of three broad attachment categories: *secure, anxious–resistant* (or *ambivalent*), and *anxious–avoidant*. (More recently researchers identified a fourth pattern, *disorganized* attachment [Main & Solomon, 1990]. Although not part of Ainsworth's original coding system [Ainsworth et al., 1978], most studies now include this pattern.)

Several studies in recent years have examined the relationship between these attachment categories and what has gone on between the infant and caregiver during the early months of life. To a large extent, quality of attachment as measured by the Ainsworth procedure seems to reflect the quality of care provided to the child thus far, particularly the sensitivity with which the caregiver has responded to the baby's cues and signals. Importantly, studies also have shown quality of attachment to be a significant predictor of the child's later adaptation and development.

Following is a description of the four major attachment categories, the behaviors that characterize each category, the caregiving behaviors that seem most likely to lead to each attachment pattern, and some of the subsequent child behaviors that have been associated with each pattern. Table 3.1 presents a brief summary of this material.

Note: The Ainsworth (Ainsworth et al., 1978) assessment procedure was developed for research purposes and has not been validated for clinical use. We believe that it is possible to support the development of strong, healthy parent–infant attachments without necessarily doing standardized assessments to classify the quality of those relationships. Nevertheless, it is important for early interventionists to be acquainted with the procedure, informed about related research, and alert to some of the "red flags" in regard to attachment.

THE SECURELY ATTACHED CHILD

The child who is securely attached plays and explores with confidence and enthusiasm in the presence of the attachment figure, periodically sharing a look, a vocalization, or a smile, or showing the caregiver a toy. The child usually is not unduly upset by the presence of a stranger as long as the caregiver is nearby. When the caregiver leaves the room briefly, the securely attached child may be very upset or may merely show a decreased interest in play. (Differences in level of distress may reflect temperament, how much experience the child has had with the caregiver leaving, or situational variables such as fatigue or not feeling well.) Regardless of the degree of visible upset during the separation episodes, the securely attached child will show clear signs of pleasure and/or relief upon the caregiver's return. If not extremely distraught, the child will greet the caregiver with a smile or a babble or perhaps

TABLE 3.1. Types of Attachments: Antecedents and Possible Consequences

	Pattern of care	Attachment behavior at age 12–18 months	Possible long-term outcomes
Secure	Sensitive, responsive	Feels secure, explores readily, accepts comfort	Confident, connected
Anxious–resistant (ambivalent)	Erratic, unpredictable	Hesitant, preoccupied with caregiver, resists comfort	Anxious, dependent
Anxious–avoidant	Unresponsive	Distant, flat affect, does not seek comfort	Aggressive, lacks empathy
Disorganized	Threatening	Confused, anxious	Dissociative

hold up a toy for the caregiver to see. If crying, the child will readily seek and accept comfort from the caregiver, and that comfort will be effective in helping the child to settle and return to play and exploration. It is clear that at this stage of the child's development, the presence of the caregiver is a significant source of security. We can expect that as the child develops, such security will become internalized so that he or she can feel confident to move further out into the world to explore and learn.

Research has shown secure attachment to grow from the child's experience with a caregiver who is consistently responsive to the child's cues and signals. This child has learned to trust that the caregiver will be there to meet his or her needs. And, importantly, this child has learned to trust in his or her own ability to solicit that care. Experience tells the child that, "When I give a signal, it counts. I have the power to see that my needs are met." That basic trust in caregivers and in self, or what sometimes is described as the child's *internal working model* (Bretherton & Waters, 1985) of self and others, is carried forward, influencing the child's expectations and behavior in subsequent relationships with other adults and peers. When these children are followed into the preschool and school years, they are found to be more cooperative, enthusiastic, persistent in problem solving, and more socially competent with their peers than children who had an insecure attachment in infancy. Although not an inoculation against later problems, secure attachment in infancy does seem to lay the foundation for healthy resolution of subsequent developmental issues (Arend, Gove, & Sroufe, 1979; Erickson, Sroufe, & Egeland, 1985; Lewis, Feiring, McGuffog, & Jaskir, 1984; Sroufe, 1983).

THE ANXIOUS–RESISTANT (OR AMBIVALENT) CHILD

This child seems preoccupied with maintaining contact with the caregiver even prior to the upsetting separation episodes in the Strange Situation procedure. The child may cling to the caregiver or check back so often that he or she never completely engages in play and exploration. It appears that the child is so unsure of the caregiver's availability and predictability that he or she dares not venture out, even within the confines of the small assessment room. Usually extremely upset by separation from the caregiver, this child nevertheless appears ambivalent during reunion, often alternating between desperate clinginess and active resistance (sometimes even aggression) when the caregiver offers comfort. The caregiver's efforts to comfort the child are not successful, and the child continues to fuss rather than going about the natural 1-year-old business of playing and learning from the world.

This pattern of attachment has been shown to be related to inconsistent, unpredictable care during the early months of the child's life
(Ainsworth et al., 1978; Egeland & Farber, 1984). Thus the child's
behavior in the Strange Situation is an understandable adaptation to a
world in which his or her signals sometimes work and sometimes do not.
The child is never sure whether others will be there to respond and care
for him or her or whether the child will be effective in soliciting the care
he or she needs. Not surprisingly, when these children are followed into
preschool and the early school years, they often lack the autonomy and
initiative we would hope to see. They are more likely to be overly
dependent on their teachers for help and attention, and they are less well
liked by their peers than are the children with a history of secure attachment (Erickson & Pianta, 1985, 1989; Erickson et al., 1985; Sroufe,
1983.)

THE ANXIOUS–AVOIDANT CHILD

This child interacts minimally, if at all, with the caregiver prior to the
separation episodes. He or she may look "precociously independent,"
playing alone with no apparent need to check to make sure the caregiver
is present, even in this unfamiliar environment. Then when the caregiver
leaves the room, this child shows no visible signs of distress. (It is interesting to note, however, that in one study, physiological measures indicated an increased arousal level among anxious–avoidant children when
their mothers left the room. Thus it has been inferred that these children
feel distress, but have already learned to block those feelings.) When the
caregiver returns to the room, anxious–avoidant children actively avoid
interaction, averting their faces or perhaps moving to the other side of
the room.

The anxious–avoidant pattern of attachment often stems from experience with a caregiver who is chronically unresponsive to the baby's
bids for care and attention. Early in life, these babies appear to be working hard to engage their caregivers. But by 1 year of age, when the
Strange Situation procedure is used, they have effectively given up. It is
almost as if they are saying, "I'm going to reject Mom before she can
reject me." Researchers also have found some parents of anxious–
avoidant babies to be intrusive and interfering, imposing their agenda on
the baby without regard to the needs and interests the baby is communicating. For example, a parent might forcefully shove the bottle in the
baby's mouth even as the baby turns away or pushes the bottle away. Or
a parent might smother the baby's face with kisses as the baby squirms
to get away.

Child care providers sometimes misread the lack of affect when

Mom or Dad drops off or picks up an anxious–avoidant infant or toddler. They may interpret this behavior as "good" and compliant, without considering the possibility that it may indicate insecure attachment. By the time these children are in preschool, they are very likely to present significant behavior problems. Teachers characterize them as either withdrawn or acting out, unpopular with their peers, lacking motivation and persistence in learning, and sometimes exhibiting unusual behaviors, such as self-stimulation or self-abuse (Erickson & Pianta, 1985, 1989; Erickson et al., 1985; Sroufe, 1983).

THE DISORGANIZED CHILD

Recent attachment research (Main & Solomon, 1990) describes a fourth pattern of attachment, often characterized as "disorganized." These children often present contradicting behaviors simultaneously, such as reaching out to the caregiver with a grimace on their face or starting to approach and then "freezing" (Main & Solomon, 1990). Although less is known about the meaning of this pattern, some researchers have found it to be associated with traumatic abuse (Cicchetti & Barnett, 1991; Main & Hesse, 1990; Crittenden, 1988). It is easy to imagine that it would be a confusing and disorganizing experience for babies if the person who is supposed to be their refuge at times of threat is also the *source* of threat. In one of the first longitudinal studies of children with disorganized attachment, University of Minnesota researchers report a high incidence of dissociative symptoms among these children in their teens (Carlson, 1998; Ogawa, Sroufe, Weinfield, Carlson, & Egeland, 1997). More research on this pattern of attachment is necessary before much can be said about the implications for intervention.

Attachment in Special Populations

In general, children are predisposed to become attached to their caregivers. Children with developmental disabilities are no exception, although the process may be more complex. It may require more time when the child's cognitive development is delayed. Or, in cases of motor or sensory impairment, children may be less adept at signaling their needs and wishes. Yet caregiver sensitivity and responsiveness remain crucial to secure attachment. Parents and other caregivers may face greater challenges in recognizing and reading the child's cues and signals, as well as in adapting their own behavior and the child's environment to elicit and support a healthy attachment process. The basic concepts in the following discussion of parental sensitivity, however, are applicable to children with special needs, as well as to children who are developing typically.

THE PATH TO SECURITY AND COMPETENCE:
PARENTAL SENSITIVITY

Given the apparent importance of secure attachment in the early months and years of life, caregivers and interventionists may ask, "What can I do about this?" Although there are no recipes that can instruct us in five easy steps to help a parent and child develop a secure attachment, we can find some guidance in the longitudinal research that examines developmental antecedents of attachment and in some intervention research that builds on that knowledge.

Sensitive care for children in the early months of life emerges as the most powerful predictor of the quality of the child's attachment (Ainsworth et al., 1978; Egeland & Farber, 1984). Parental sensitivity and responsiveness also are associated with a higher level of mastery motivation (Yarrow, Rubenstein, & Pederson, 1975) and higher intellectual functioning at subsequent ages (Beckwith, Cohen, Kopp, Parmelee, & Marcy, 1976; Bradley & Caldwell, 1984). At the other end of the spectrum, insensitivity has been described as the common thread among the various patterns of child maltreatment. Whether a child is physically abused, verbally abused, or physically or emotionally neglected, the underlying insensitivity appears to be the central factor accounting for long-term psychological consequences (Erickson & Egeland, 1987; Erickson, Egeland, & Pianta, 1989). Thus promoting parental sensitivity becomes a logical target of early intervention efforts.

Although sensitivity is a commonly used word, it may connote different things to different people. Therefore, it is important to begin with a clear operational definition as used in the child development research literature. *Sensitivity*, as developmental researchers define it, encompasses (1) recognizing the infant's ability to signal needs, (2) accurately reading and interpreting cues, (3) responding contingently, and (4) responding consistently and predictably.

First of all, sensitivity implies a recognition that even the youngest infant can signal his or her needs and wishes. That may sound simple and self-evident; however, not all parents recognize the remarkable communication capabilities of a newborn baby. Some parents may think of the baby as an object or a tiny doll to dress up, feed, and cuddle according to an adult timetable. They may be unaware that even in the first days of life, the baby is a human being with needs and wishes and the ability to communicate those needs and wishes through a wide range of facial expressions, gestures, postures, and different kinds of cries.

In our own work, we have found that it is useful to begin even before the baby is born to help the parents think of the baby as a human being with his or her own characteristics and preferences. For example, in the Steps Toward Effective, Enjoyable Parenting (STEEP) program (Egeland & Erickson, 1990; Erickson, 1989; Erickson et al., 1992), we encourage the expectant parents to pay attention to the activity level of their baby in utero at different times of day or in different circumstances (e.g., when Mom is trying to sleep, after Mom eats certain foods, when there is a lot of noise in the house, or when Mom is very active). This simple exercise can help lay the foundation for understanding the reciprocal nature of the parent–child relationship, that what the parent does influences the child and vice versa.

Once the baby arrives, it is helpful to direct the parents' attention to how the newborn responds to his or her surroundings. It's thrilling to discover how the baby turns toward Mom's familiar voice, shuts out loud noises and goes to sleep, or finds his or her thumb to suck when needing comfort.

Secondly, sensitivity involves accurate reading and interpretation of the baby's cues and signals. An excellent resource for parents who want to learn about the meaning of their baby's signals is Born Dancing by Thoman and Browder (1987), described in the annotated list of resources in the Appendix at the end of this book. Also, as a resource for work with parents of infants, we present in Table 3.2 a list of many of the common signals that babies give to indicate that they want to engage in interaction or that they want to disengage. This list was adapted from the work of Kathryn Barnard, a pioneer in home visiting for new parents and a primary developer of the Nursing Child Assessment Satellite Training Programs (NCAST) system of parent–child observation, in which many public health nurses around the country have been trained (Barnard, 1979). As described later in this chapter, guided viewing of videotapes of parent–child interaction is an especially valuable strategy for building on parents' ability to interpret their baby's individual style of communicating.

The hallmark of sensitivity is that the adult's response is contingent on the baby's signals. This means that the parent takes the baby's cries seriously and responds accordingly by providing comfort. Likewise, the parent cuddles the baby when the baby gives signals that say cuddling feels good. The parent also allows the baby quiet time without stimulation when the baby's cues seem to say, "Leave me alone." When working with parents we often describe this sensitive, synchronous interaction as being "like slow dancing with your baby and letting the baby lead." Of course, there are plenty of times when parents will need to be in charge and set the schedule, especially as the child becomes old enough to be taught the rules and expectations of fitting into a social world. But research indicates that in the early months of life, it is beneficial for the

TABLE 3.2. Definitions of Infant Cues

I.   Subtle engagement cues

    A. Alerting—Increased muscle tone of face, possibly with flushing to cheeks, eyes usually sparkle.

    B. Brow raising—Elevating of eyebrows and formation of horizontal lines in forehead.

    C. Feeding posture—Moderate abduction of the lower arms, forearm flexion, and fisted hands held palm inward.

    D. Head raising—Elevation of head with eyes directed upward toward caregiver.

II. Potent engagement cues

    A. Facing gaze—Looking at the parent's face.

    B. Mutual gaze—Sustained eye-to-eye contact.

III. Subtle disengagement cues

    A. Facial grimace—Combination of a frown, eye tightening, and upper lip raising.

    B. Eyes clinched—Eyes tightly shut.

    C. Gaze aversion—Eyes turned away from caregiver or object.

    D. Diffuse body movements—Motor movement of arms and legs, usually tight or close in toward torso; movements can be jerky and give the impression that infant is struggling.

    E. Immobility—Can be either positive or disengagement cue; a stilling of movement of arms or legs, as if in anticipation of something to come.

    F. Head lowering—Chin brought in toward chest, eyes usually lowered as well.

    G. Hand to ear, neck, or behind neck—Self-explanatory, a tonic neck reflex related behavior.

IV. Potent disengagement cues

    A. Crying (three types)

        1. Hunger or ordinary cry: somewhat low in volume, of short duration (1–2 seconds); rhythmical, with vocalization and 1–2 second pause, vocalization and 1–2 second pause, and so forth.

        2. Angry cry: a more forceful version of the hunger or ordinary cry, remains rhythmical.

        3. Pain cry: a vocalization of sudden onset, of long duration (approximately 7 seconds); loud, followed by audible expelling of air, gulping in air, repetition of above.

    B. Whining—A prolonged, high-pitched, somewhat nasal sound; not rhythmical, uttered by itself and repeated a few times in succession.

    C. Fussing—Staccato, short, low-pitched vocalizations; not rhythmical.

    D. Spitting—Eructations of small amounts of food, without gagging or forceful projection.

(Continued on next page)

TABLE 3.2. *continued*

E. Pulling away—Removing torso and/or head away from caregiver or object; that is, withdrawing and increasing distance from caregiver or object.

F. Tray pound—Hitting the surface of high chair tray or table top with the palm of the hand.

G. Lateral head shake—Turning head from side to side as if saying no.

Note. Partial list of infant cues obtained from Sumner and Spietz (1994). Copyright 1994 by NCAST Publications. Reprinted by permission.

baby to have the experience of "driving" the interaction with parents. That experience allows the baby to begin to develop confidence that others will respond and, reciprocally, that he or she is able to get a response when needed.

Finally, sensitivity implies consistency and predictability over time. As described in the previous section on secure parent–child attachment, consistent, predictable care demonstrates to children that they can count on others to be there. It also demonstrates that children have some power to influence others, to seek actively and effectively to have their needs met. Of course, no parent can or should jump at every little signal a baby gives. But infants' overall experiences—the sum or average of all of their bids for attention and expressions of need—should be that their signals work and that caregivers are available and willing to respond.

Indications of Parental Insensitivity

Insensitivity may be manifest in various ways. It sometimes is a *persistent, chronic failure to respond* to the infant's cries and other bids for attention, which is an especially pernicious form of insensitivity. The long-term effects of emotional unresponsiveness have been shown to include anxious–avoidant attachment, declining intellectual functioning, and serious behavior problems (Egeland & Erickson, 1987; Erickson & Egeland, 1987, 1996; Erickson et al., 1989). In fact, those studies indicate that emotional neglect, at least in the first 2 years of life, may do even more long-term psychological harm to a child than other, more overt types of maltreatment. In its most extreme form, emotional neglect results in "failure to thrive," which often ends in death.

When a caregiver is unresponsive to the child's signals, that does not necessarily mean that there is an absence of interaction with the child. Rather, it means that interactions are driven by the adult's agenda instead of being contingent on the needs and wishes of the child. For example, a father may occasionally cuddle or play with the child when the mood strikes him, but ignore the child's attempts to initiate such interactions. Parents who are emotionally unresponsive may not look neglectful in other ways. They may dress the child in nice clothes, feed him, attend to his basic health care needs, and provide a clean, physically safe home. Yet they do not attend to the child's bids for comfort and/or stimulation.

Insensitivity is sometimes manifest in inconsistent, erratic patterns of responding. One day the parent is highly attentive to the child's cues, but the next day seems wrapped up in other things and disregards the child's signals. Over time, the child does not know what to expect, unsure of the availability of the parent and unsure of his or her own ability to solicit needed care and attention. Of course, there will be fluctuations from day to day, or hour to hour, in the life of any family, and no parent can or should be hovering over a child watching for every tiny cue. We are talking here about significant and frequent lapses in the emotional availability of the parent, major and cumulative lapses that will have a significant impact on how the child views others and self.

Another form of insensitivity is intrusiveness, in which interactions are driven by the adult's needs and wishes, despite the fact that the child's signals say that he or she needs or wants something different. For example, intrusiveness is sometimes a failure to recognize or respect the child's signals that say, "I don't feel like playing (or eating or being tickled or kissed) right now." The caregiver may respond when the child initiates interaction, providing comfort, attention, and stimulation when the child signals such needs. But then when the child signals that he or she has had enough, the caregiver continues to keep the interaction going. Intrusiveness may instead involve the caregiver interfering with the child's self-directed play and exploration. For example, in a recent parenting group we watched one mother repeatedly try to "teach" her baby to stack rings on a post, while the baby was far more interested in making noise by banging two of the rings together. Whereas one such episode may be innocuous, a persistent pattern of trying to direct the child's activity without regard for the child's own wishes is cause for concern.

It is important to note that sensitivity is an issue not only for parents, but for all of us who work with children. In fact, as early intervention professionals, we sometimes are the worst offenders in terms of intrusiveness. For example, we may persistently try to engage an infant in developmentally stimulating activities even when the child's behavior clearly tells us that this is not the time. If we allow ourselves to be driven only by what is on our "lesson plan" for the day, rather than by the baby's cues, we are missing a wonderful opportunity to give the child a message that his or her wishes count. And we forego an excellent chance to reinforce for the parent how important it is to read and respect the child's signals.

Keep in mind that insensitivity does not imply bad intentions on the part of the adult. Insensitivity may result from inaccurate knowledge and erroneous beliefs about child development (e.g., that responding consistently to a baby's cries will "spoil" the baby); stress and exhaustion that sap the parent of the energy necessary to stay attuned to the child's cues; or emotional issues that render the caregiver unable to be emotionally available to the child. A parent's capacity to respond sensitively requires an awareness of the meaning of cues and signals, a willingness to respond, and the emotional strength and social support necessary to sustain sensitivity over time (Dunst & Trivette, 1990). Each of these factors associated with sensitivity can be addressed within the context of our early intervention partnership with parents. (Some of the issues that underlie sensitivity are discussed in the next two chapters of this book.)

USING VIDEOTAPING AND GUIDED VIEWING TO ENHANCE SENSITIVITY

One of the most promising strategies for enhancing parental sensitivity involves videotaping parent–child interactions, then watching the tape and discussing it with the parents.

In the STEEP program (Egeland & Erickson, 1990; Erickson et al., 1992), we have used videotaping extensively with new parents and their babies, and parents report it to be one of the most useful and enjoyable aspects of the program. We give the tape to the parents when they graduate from the program, an incentive that many mothers say drew them to the program in the first place. Our approach to using videotaping, as described in an education video *Seeing Is Believing* (Erickson, 1999), has now been adopted by several other early intervention programs working with a variety of children and families, including researchers in the Netherlands who report success in using this as a short-term strategy with moderately at-risk parents (Bakermans-Kranenburg & Juffer, 1996). These strategies also reportedly are very helpful in interpreting the meaning of signals provided by infants with developmental disabilities, whose cues often are less vigorous or clear than those of a more robust baby.

Why Videotape?

In times of limited resources, especially money, the idea of purchasing video equipment seems unrealistic for some agencies. However, we are convinced that the benefits outweigh the cost. We see the advantages of videotaping to be as follows:

1. *Videotaping promotes self-evaluation and self-affirmation.* Rather than defining ourselves as "judges" of the parent's behavior, we engage the parent in a process of self-reflection. Videotape affords some distance, allowing parents to step back, watch more objectively, and react somewhat as critics viewing a movie.

2. *Videotaping recognizes the parent as the expert on his or her own child.* Viewing techniques discussed later use open-ended questions to facilitate parents' observation and identification of their child's behavior.

3. *Videotaping focuses on strengths, both for parent and child.* Through focusing questions and observations on visible strengths, we set a positive tone for the viewing, discussion, and overall interaction with a family.

4. *Videotaping provides a permanent record for monitoring change.* Videotapes provide visual and auditory evidence of change in parent–child behaviors and interactions over time. This allows parents to discover how they're building parenting skills, and it is invaluable to family workers and supervisors as a record of progress.

5. *Videotaping personifies the infant.* Parents who may have perceived their baby as an inanimate little doll can recognize that the baby is a living human being with unique characteristics and feelings.

6. *Videotaping promotes perspective taking.* When parents view their baby's physical response to an incident on screen, they can more easily understand the baby's point of view and practice taking his or her perspective in future interactions.

7. *Videotaping affirms the individuality of the child.* Watching their infant in action on screen intensifies parents' perception of that baby as a separate and unique individual. Rather than a generalized view of what 3-month-old babies do, the focus is on what *this* 3-month-old does. This can be especially important when a baby's development is atypical.

8. *Videotaping conveys the notion of reciprocity, of mutual influence.* Witnessing the give and take during a routine occurrence such as diapering helps parents comprehend the complementary influence of parent on baby and baby on parent.

9. *Videotaping engages the extended family and friends in intervention.* When able to watch a parent and baby on video over time, extended family members and friends often become interested and involved in the intervention process.

In general, using videotaping and discussion with parents is an excellent strategy for helping them become better observers of their children, an essential component of parental sensitivity to cues and signals. Additionally, as a permanent record of behavior, videotape is useful to staff and supervisors for identifying strengths in both parent and child and for monitoring progress. And if parents and front-line staff feel overwhelmed by the challenges the child and family face, another colleague or supervisor with more distance from the situation can look at the tape and see the strengths more easily and clearly.

Setting It Up

Videotaping can be done in the home, at the clinic, in a classroom, or at the neighborhood park, depending on what is most comfortable for the family and what works for us within the parameters of our work setting. It is important that we let the parents know right away that we are not there to judge or scrutinize what they are doing. We are there instead to enable them to see for themselves what is happening with them and their child. We want them to have a chance to step outside of their relationship with their child to see more clearly the special strengths and characteristics that they and their child bring to their interactions. And we want to work with them to build on those strengths, to make the most of their time with their child.

We have found it useful to videotape routine kinds of child care tasks, such as feeding, diapering, or bathing (a wonderfully rich opportunity to observe infant cues and the caregiver's adaptation to those signals!). Often we videotape parents and children playing together, sometimes asking them to do what they and their child most enjoy. Or we may say, "What new things is your child doing these days? How might we set up a situation so that we are likely to see his or her new accomplishments?" (Note that we do not suggest that the parent "try to get him to do it," but rather that we set up a situation where it might happen naturally. This is consistent with our emphasis on letting the child lead the interaction.) Often we will introduce a new, age-appropriate toy and suggest that the parent see how the child responds to it, in the spirit of exploring together the child's changing interests and skills.

It is common for parents to feel self-conscious the first few times they are videotaped, perhaps focusing primarily on how they look or sound on tape. But as they become accustomed to seeing themselves on the video screen, they begin to relax and become more natural, usually shifting their focus more to the child and their interactions with him or her. It is a good idea to videotape quite frequently at first, in order to get over the initial awkwardness and get down to the business (and fun) of learning through this technique.

Watching and Learning Together

It is ideal to view the tape with the parent immediately after taping. Most portable cameras will function as a VCR by using a small cable to connect them to the back of a regular TV, so even if the family does not have a VCR you should be able to view the tape in the home. (You probably will want to practice with the camera and your own TV before you try this with a family. In our experience, the biggest obstacle to using guided viewing of videotapes with families seems to be the discomfort of professionals in using the equipment. We call it "techno-phobia"! Most equipment really is quite simple to use if you practice and then put simple instructions inside the case as a reminder to yourself.) If it is not possible to watch the tape right away, or if you cannot watch it at all on equipment available in the home, it is important to decide right away when and where to watch and discuss it with the parent.

When we view a videotape with parents, we do it as "co-investigators" or "partners in the journey," working together to figure out how the baby communicates his or her needs and wishes, what new things he or she is doing or trying to do, and, in general, what this baby's style and preferences are at this point in development. Consistent with a strength-focused, empowerment approach, this strategy helps parents identify and build on their own knowledge and skills rather than setting up the professional as the "expert" who teaches parents how to respond.

We have found it to be most productive and nonthreatening to view the tape privately with the family, rather than watching it in a class or group. Self-consciousness and a sense of competitiveness among parents can stand in the way of effective use of the tapes in a group. However, it is sometimes efficient and worthwhile to videotape a parent and child when they are in a group setting, and then view the tape alone with the parent at a later time.

The following is an exercise in preparing to use videotaping as we describe above.

1. Watch a 10- to 15-minute videotape of a parent and child interacting with each other.
2. On a sheet of paper, write down all the strengths observed in the child.
3. Next, write down all the strengths observed in the parent.
4. Only after noting the strengths, write down anything that could be done differently in this interaction.
5. Write down several open-ended questions or observations to address with this parent while viewing the tape together. Comments should:
   a. Be nonjudgmental,

b. Be nondirective, and

c. Lead the parent to discover and own the knowledge.

Table 3.3 presents a list of some of the questions and comments typical of those we have found to be most effective as we view tapes with families, and can be applied freely to the exercise above. Although we go out of our way to recognize the expertise of parents and to avoid setting ourselves up as the ones with the answers, sometimes parents will respond to a question in a way that is clearly incorrect or not appropriate. For example, they may make an observation that is grounded in inaccurate knowledge of child development or reflects an unrealistic interpretation of what is going on with the baby. Rather than refuting the parent's beliefs directly, we have found that it works well to say something like "That doesn't quite fit with what I've been taught about babies, but I wonder where we could get more information about that." This provides an opportunity to encourage the parent's quest for knowledge and to reinforce the use of resource materials by gathering relevant

TABLE 3.3. Using Videotaping to Promote Parental Sensitivity, by Martha Farrell Erickson, PhD

Try to videotape the parent and infant in natural situations such as feeding, bathing, diaper changing, and play. A good way to lead into taping play situations, which are sometimes more threatening to the parent than more concrete tasks, is to ask the parent to show you some of the things the baby enjoys. If the parent doesn't know what to do, you might provide an age-appropriate toy and lead the parent in trying to discover such things as how the baby visually tracks objects, whether the baby is reaching for things, how he or she responds to sounds, whether the baby shows a visual preference for some things (including Mom's face) over others, and so forth. After taping, view the tape with the parent, using the following as a guide for discussion.

I.   Suggested questions to ask the parent as you view the tape (push the pause button when you want to focus on a specific behavior)

    A. "You seemed to know just what he or she wanted there. How could you tell?"

    B. "What do you think your baby was feeling then?"

    C. "How did your baby communicate his or her feelings there? (More generally, how *does* your baby communicate to you?)"

    D. "Look at what your baby just did (pointing out some expression, gesture, posture, etc.). What do you think he or she was trying to tell you?" (If you know the parent is reading signal incorrectly, say, "Maybe so. Often, though, when babies do that it means. . . . ")

    E. "I wonder how it feels to a baby when. . . . " (pointing out specific parental behavior, such as tossing in air, gentle stroking, etc.).

(Continued on next page)

TABLE 3.3. *continued*

F. "What kinds of things do/did *you* like to hear, see, feel, experience (now or as a child)?" (Use parent's own feelings to lead to perspective taking about how the baby experiences things. For example, "It sure feels good to be cuddled, doesn't it? I bet your baby likes that feeling too.")

G. "When people see themselves on video, they sometimes feel critical of the way they look, sound, act. Is there anything you see that you'd like to change about what you did on the video?" (Explore in a supportive way.)

H. Either while watching the videotape or watching live parent–infant interaction, it sometimes is helpful to "talk through" the baby. For example, "Hey Mom, I like to look at your face," or "Ooh, I feel scared when I get tossed around so much."

II. Some things to watch and listen for in tapes of parent–infant interaction

    A. Tone of voice, choice of words when talking to baby.

    B. Distance between parent's face and baby's (babies love to look at faces, but can't focus if the face is too close or too far).

    C. Unsolicited kissing or prolonged mouth kissing, a common form of intrusiveness (perhaps can be redirected to gentle kissing on top of head or cheek); cuddling when baby is tired and/or seeking cuddling, but not when baby signals desire to explore and play.

    D. Tossing around or overzealous swinging or roughhousing.

    E. Misreading startle response as pleasure (relates to D above).

    F. Moving objects in front of baby too quickly for him or her to focus on.

    G. Failure to read baby's signals that say "leave me alone" (e.g., continuing to try to feed or play with baby when baby does not want to).

    H. "Teasing" baby with bottle or toys (e.g., pulling bottle out of mouth to see baby's reaction; holding toy out for baby, then pulling it away as he or she attempts to grab it). (*Note:* An important message for parents is that the baby needs opportunities to learn that he or she can signal needs and make successful efforts.)

    I. Attributing too much intentionality to baby (e.g., "He or she is trying to get back at me").

---

materials from the library or calling an information line. This also presents a clear, affirming message to the parent that he or she can check out these kinds of things whether or not we are around.

Recognizing Parent Strengths

As we view videotapes with parents and interact with families in our centers and their homes, we want to keep our focus on the strong points of parent–child interaction. To accomplish this, we will need to use our observation skills, that is, to *pay attention* and really watch and *see* what is going on between parent and infant. *Seeing* means looking beyond the behaviors we observe to consider possible meanings or motivations for these behaviors.

Then, for example, during ordinary moments such as feeding, we may observe that the infant is closely watching her father's face and we can comment, "Your baby sure keeps a close eye on you—she must think a lot of you." To a mother who has brought along a bag of crackers and a few toys to the waiting room for her active toddler, we can say, "Looks like you were planning ahead."

BEYOND ATTACHMENT: CRITICAL PARENTING BEHAVIORS FOR OPTIMAL LEARNING AND DEVELOPMENT

Based on a comprehensive review of the literature, Ramey and Ramey (1992) identify six elements of children's environments that facilitate development. They call them "essential daily ingredients" (p. 342). Interventionists, caregivers, and parents can work together to supply these ingredients in the lives of all infants and toddlers. To promote cognitive development and good attitudes toward learning, all children need the following:

1. *Encouragement of exploration.* To be encouraged by adults to explore and to gather information about their environments.
2. *Mentoring in basic skills.* To be mentored by trusted adults in basic cognitive skills, such as labeling, sorting, sequencing, comparing, and noting means–ends relations.
3. *Celebration of developmental advances.* To have their developmental accomplishments celebrated and reinforced by people with whom they spend a lot of time.
4. *Guided rehearsal and extension of new skills.* To have others help them in rehearsing and then elaborating upon and extending their newly acquired skills.
5. *Protection from inappropriate disapproval, teasing, or punishment.* To avoid negative experiences associated with adults' disapproval, teasing, or punishment for those behaviors that are normal and necessary in children's trial-and-error learning about their environments.
6. *Provision of a rich and responsive language environment.* To have adults provide a predictable and comprehensible communication environment, in which language is used to convey infor-

mation, provide social rewards, and encourage learning of new materials and skills. (Ramey & Ramey, 1992, pp. 342–344)

In the following sections, we elaborate on elements that are especially relevant during the infant and toddler periods. For a detailed discussion of the "essential daily ingredients," see Ramey and Ramey (1999) in the resource bibliography at the end of the book.

Baby Talk: Facilitating Language Development, Building Memories

How parents talk to their babies and toddlers is an especially critical parental behavior to consider in early intervention, even long before children develop the ability to speak. Sometimes parents do not recognize the need to talk to a baby who is too young to understand spoken language. For example, a number of studies have shown that teen mothers talk less to their babies than older mothers (e.g., Epstein, 1980; Osofsky & Osofsky, 1970). Recently, Hart and Risley (1995) documented striking differences in early language experiences among groups of middle-class families, low-income families, and families on welfare. Some parents may give up talking if their baby initially is unresponsive to their talk, as may occur with infants with developmental disabilities. It may sometimes be necessary to help parents develop a rationale for talking to their babies. The most obvious reason is that talking to babies, long before they can understand the words or talk back, has been shown to be a factor in promoting language development and later learning (Clarke-Stewart, 1973; Hart & Risley, 1995). The Hart and Risley study showed that sheer quantity of early language exposure accounted for later differences between middle-class and low-income children.

New neuroscientific findings suggest that early language exposure actually affects the structures of the brain, which in turn allow effective acquisition and transmission of information. Recent research on brain development suggests that at birth, a baby's brain contains 100 billion neurons. Starting shortly after birth, the brain produces trillions more connections among neurons than it can possibly use. Connections that are used through a baby's experiences with the people and objects in his or her environment remain; connections that are unused are eliminated. By 6 months of age, an infant can recognize and produce the vowel sounds that are common to the language of his caregiver. By age 10 years or sooner, excess connections are dramatically pruned, and patterns of emotion and thought are formed characteristic to that child (Begley, 1996; Greenough, Black, & Wallace, 1987; Nash, 1997; Shore, 1997).

When a baby begins to babble and experiment with his or her own voice, parents can reinforce the babbling by imitating the baby's sounds and engaging in a reciprocal "conversation" with the baby. Mothers and fathers from many cultures often use a peculiar form of talk called *parentese*. Infants' heart rates increase and their word–object recognition is accelerated when parents put their faces close to the child and speak slowly in short sentences with a high pitched, musical voice (Shore, 1997). This interplay is an important lesson for the baby in language, as well as in cause and effect.

How parents talk with their babies also has value in the arena of social and emotional development. The parent's voice is an important source of comfort for a baby (Nugent, 1985). What a relief for parents, struggling to stay on top of other tasks while still caring for a baby, to discover that their baby can be comforted just by the sound of a familiar voice rather than always needing to be picked up or fed! In contrast, voices sometimes can be frightening too and can undermine a child's sense of safety.

One strategy that we have used to address a variety of issues with families involves writing letters to the parents as if we were their baby talking to them. (In Chapter 4, we will discuss the value of this strategy in promoting perspective taking.) The letter presented in Table 3.4 is one that encouraged many parents to stop and think about the importance of how they talk to their babies.

Talking gently, playfully, and positively to babies is a way of establishing habits for when the child is older. In our work, we have found this "practice" time to be important for parents who have a coarse, rough way of talking with friends and family. For example, upon hearing herself on videotape with her new baby, one mother said, "Oh, no! Do I always talk in that 'whiskey baritone'?"

Hart and Risley (1995) also identify quality features of language and interaction that enhance children's development. They include the following:

1. *Language diversity.* The more often a child hears a parent use words in relation to a variety of events and experiences, the more varied and refined are the meanings of words for the child.
2. *Feedback tone.* Positive feedback is described as parent repetitions, extensions, expansions of child utterances; confirmations; praise; or approval. Negative feedback includes imperatives to warn or prohibit, disconfirmations, criticisms, or disparagements.
3. *Symbolic emphasis.* Parents emphasize what the culture expects children to notice, name, recall, and relate to other words and

TABLE 3.4. Sample "Letter from Baby," by Martha Farrell Erickson, PhD

Dear Mommy and Daddy,

I've been noticing something interesting lately. Even though I don't know how to talk yet, or even understand the words you say to me, sometimes I get a really good feeling when you talk to me. Your voice sounds happy and full of love, and it gives me the same warm feeling I get when you cuddle me. Even if you're busy cooking or cleaning and can't pick me up, I feel great hearing you say my name and tell me things. Listening to you talk makes it easier for me to wait until you're done with your work and can hold me or play with me. It's especially fun when you make silly sounds or sing songs to me. I don't even mind if you're off-key or mess up the words! Hearing you helps to entertain me and keeps me from feeling bored.

Sometimes voices make me feel bad, too. Even though I don't know the meaning of the words, sometimes voices sound angry or scary. Then, I feel kind of jittery and start to cry. When voices are loud or angry, it's hard for me to feel calm and safe and loved. (You probably know what I mean, 'cause I bet you've had those feelings, too, when people talked in a way that was scary to you.)

I've already figured out that almost everyone uses an angry voice some of the time, but I'm glad that most of the time you talk to me in a nice, gentle voice. If I keep listening to you and other people talk, pretty soon I'll start to understand what the words mean, and I'll even figure out how to talk myself—just like you. In fact, when I do start talking, I bet you'll be really glad that you've talked so nicely to me, because the way I talk will be the same way that I hear you talk. I wonder what my first words will be? Maybe Mama or Dada? Someday, I can even use words to tell you I love you, but for now I'll just have to tell you with my smiles and hugs. OK?

Love,

(Baby's Name)

experiences in speaking and thinking. Using a lot of nouns, modifiers, and past-tense verbs emphasizes these relations between things and events.

4. *Guidance style.* How often the child is asked rather than told what to do is exemplified by preceding prompts with phrases such as "Can you . . . ? Do you . . . ? Shall we . . . ?", rather than giving plain, directive statements.

5. *Responsiveness.* This denotes the relative amount of a child's experience with controlling the course of interaction. Parents show an interest in supporting and encouraging a child's lan-

guage practice and an appreciation of a child's skill level and choice of topic. (pp. 150–154)

Of course the content of parental talk is important as well, even before the baby is mature enough to comprehend the words. What parents say to their babies is a way of building a storehouse of memories for later. Older children like to know what pet names their parents called them, what songs were sung to them, what stories they were told. Parents may recognize the importance of this if they are asked about what pet names their own parents called them, what songs and stories their parents sang or told them, and the manner in which their parents usually spoke to them. From the first day of a child's life, parents can begin to communicate their love and nurture their child's strong sense of self by the words they use and the tone of their voice.

> *The impact of what I (M.F.E.) said (and sang) to my own daughter was brought home to me in a striking way a few years ago. When Erin was a baby, I often comforted her with a silly little song I made up, "Little Erin, I love you. Little Erin, do you love me too? You're the sweetest girl I know, and I love you so!" And so on. . . . Over the years the song faded from memory as we moved on to more grown-up pursuits. But, one evening when Erin was 11, she and I were working together in the nursery during a special evening out for moms in the STEEP program. One baby was especially fussy, and I was trying everything in the book to get her to settle down. As I paced the floor with her, I unconsciously was humming the tune to the little song I used to sing for Erin. As Erin recognized the old tune, she told me in no uncertain terms, "Oh, Mom, don't sing that to her! That's my song!"*

Story Time for Baby

Reading to babies and toddlers is an excellent way for parents and caregivers to promote language learning and lay the foundation for later literacy. Especially in children's first and second years, it is another way to talk to them. In Hart and Risley's (1995) terms, positive feedback such as repetitions, extensions, expansions, confirmations, praise, and approval for child utterances are facilitated by paging through a simple children's book together. The benefits of reading to very young children are well documented (Butler, 1980; Goodman, 1986; Jalongo, 1990; Taylor, 1983). In addition to promoting language development, reading to children enhances their visual and auditory skills, reinforces basic concepts, stimulates their imagination, offers opportunities for new experiences, and serves as a prime time for snuggling and close physical contact (Kupetz & Green, 1997).

Local public libraries are usually wonderful places for parents to find a variety of appropriate books for young children, especially with the assistance of a children's or reference librarian. Taking our parent groups on field trips with their children is an effective way of introducing the public library to families who are not familiar with using it and updating others on its resources. Often libraries offer story hours for children. But if infants and toddlers are too wiggly to enjoy these scheduled group times, it's no reason for parents and caregivers to be discouraged from reading to them. Having sturdy board books (available at libraries and bookstores) on hand enables very young children to initiate the reading activity with their caregivers in the more informal setting of home or child care.

Kupetz and Green (1997) offer detailed and practical suggestions for infant and toddler book selection and guidelines for reading. Foremost among these guidelines are reading only one on one or in very small groups; positioning children so the book's pictures are easily seen; allowing children to assist in turning pages; pointing to and identifying pictures while reading; using a quiet, soft voice with animation; and reacting positively to all of children's attempts to name objects or verbalize in any way. Adults need not feel compelled to read even simple books verbatim to children. Sometimes just pointing to the pictures and talking about them is easier and more enjoyable.

As always, it's important to tune into the child's cues and signals. If a child is arching his or her back, averting his or her face, or crying, stop immediately. Reading aloud should and can be fun for both children and adults. Despite our best efforts, some infants, because of temperament or developmental delay, do not enjoy reading books until they are 1 or 2, or older. But if books are available, and adults offer the experience frequently and model their own joy of reading, most young children eventually will respond to reading with great enthusiasm.

For parents whose own literacy skills are limited, reading with their infant or toddler can be an important step toward their own educational goals. Adult literacy programs have successfully used children's books for improving adult reading skills. Children's literature also can be used as a framework for discussion on developmental issues in parent education groups. Both of these applications can help parents increase their ease and enjoyment of reading for their own purposes, as well as teach parents techniques for selecting and reading books to their children. Because the field of children's literature has rapidly expanded over the past 20 years, there is a wide and excellent selection of multicultural children's books from which to choose.

MOVING OUT INTO THE WORLD:
EXPLORATION, MASTERY, AND AUTONOMY

Essential to all aspects of the child's development is the opportunity to explore the object world. The parent's role in supporting and facilitating that exploration is critical. Studies have shown a relationship between school success and opportunities during infancy to play with a variety of materials in a relatively unrestricted physical environment (e.g., Bradley & Caldwell, 1984). This is an important issue for early intervention in some so-called high-risk families where opportunities for exploration may be impeded either by crowded, unsafe physical environments or by overly restrictive, authoritarian child-rearing practices that fail to recognize the importance of exploration for the child's development. Interventionists may need to address baby proofing the environment, providing appropriate play things at little or no cost, and expanding parental beliefs and attitudes about play and exploration.

For children with disabilities, the opportunity to explore is also crucial, but these children and their families encounter special challenges. For example, children with motor impairment or low muscle tone may be motivated to explore, but unable to act on that motivation. Parents and professionals can engage in collaborative problem solving to find ways to adapt the environment or to provide support and assistance that enable the child to explore. Williamson (1988) clearly describes, and illustrates with photographs, such a process in his case study of Allison, a 7-month-old infant with Down syndrome who exhibited passive behavior related to low muscle tone and lack of postural control. By providing various kinds of postural support to Allison, capitalizing on her visual and auditory interest in social interaction, and gradually increasing demands for motor control, Williamson together with Allison's parents successfully facilitated her development of self-initiated exploratory play.

Children not only need to explore the environment, but to master it. Infants need experiences that allow them to feel some degree of control over the environment (e.g., MacTurk, McCarthy, Vietze, & Yarrow, 1987; MacTurk, Vietze, McCarthy, McQuiston, & Yarrow, 1985). Mastery of the environment begins with the child's experience in using a cry, a smile, or outstretched arms actively to solicit a response from caregivers. As infants develop cognitive and motor skills that enable them purposefully to explore objects, mastery becomes increasingly important. The task for parents is to create situations where a goal is attainable with some effort on the part of the child.

For example, with a toy just out of reach a baby can scoot across the floor, grasp the toy, and begin to play with it. If the toy is too far out of reach, the baby will tire and give up out of frustration. On the other hand, if the parent places the toy in the baby's hand, the child is deprived of the experience of pursuing and reaching the goal. Cause-and-effect toys (e.g., squeak toys, busy boxes, Jack-in-the-boxes) are important in this period of development, certainly in terms of the child's cognitive understanding of concepts of cause and effect (Piaget, 1952), but also because of the opportunity for children to have the empowering experience of seeing their own actions bring about a consequence.

Striking a balance between giving too much help or too little help is a challenge that increases in importance as the child moves into the toddler phase when autonomy is the central developmental issue (Erikson, 1963). Parent–child difficulties around autonomy issues at age 2 have been associated with behavior problems at age 5 (Erickson, 1984; Erickson et al., 1985). Given too little help and emotional support when faced with the many problem-solving tasks that toddlers encounter each day, children feel overwhelmed and learn both that they are incompetent and that others are unavailable to help. With too much help, children get the message that others have to solve the problem because they themselves are incapable. A delicate balance is required for toddlers to experience both their own competence and the reliability of help and support when they have exhausted their own resources.

Interestingly, this parallels the experience between professional service providers and parents. Just as professionals want parents to provide just enough of a platform that children feel they have accomplished something independently, so should professionals offer only as much help or support as parents truly need. Empowerment is a central theme at all levels in family-focused intervention. When we speak of empowerment, we do not mean giving others power—as if it is ours to give. We mean supporting them in claiming their own power.

Respecting and encouraging autonomy can be especially difficult for parents of a young child with disabilities. One mother, whose daughter has limited use of her legs, tells the poignant story of watching through tears as her little girl walked slowly, with braces and crutches, to get some cookies. This mother knew how much easier it would have been to get the cookies for her daughter, but she was wise enough to cheer the girl on as she did it herself.

LIMIT SETTING AND BEHAVIOR GUIDANCE

No discussion of parenting would be complete without addressing limits and discipline. To survive in a social world, young children must begin to learn acceptable social behaviors. Parents and caregivers can teach these behaviors while supporting the toddler's sense of autonomy and mastery. The following strategies are especially effective for this process:

- *Childproof children's environments.* One of the most essential and basic strategies to promote children's autonomy and mastery is to remove delicate and breakable objects (this will not be forever, just until children are old enough to handle them safely); block access to stairways, exterior doors, and electrical outlets; keep cleaning and gardening supplies and other poisonous items inaccessible; and supervise toddlers closely at all times, especially in kitchens, bathrooms, garages, and other potentially dangerous areas. (See Green, 1994, in the resource bibliography at the end of the book for specific suggestions.) As part of redesigning environments for children, parents can pack away out-of-season or off-sized clothing and keep appropriate clothes accessible, arrange low bookshelves with books and baskets of toys, and keep a low-wattage nightlight in children's rooms. With these efforts, caregivers provide freedom of movement for children and safe opportunities for exploration.

- *Create and use routines.* Because toddlers don't understand the adult concept of time and lack the ability and experience to predict what will happen next, routines for bedtime, nap time, and life in general can be very helpful to them. For example, a bedtime routine can include a bath, reading storybooks, and a lullaby sung by a parent or a recording, with the process beginning at the same general time each night. This sequence of events will be predictable and comforting to young children and can make bedtime a pleasant time instead of an exhausting battle.

- *Use clear language.* Very young children have limited vocabularies and are extremely literal. They do not understand sarcasm or double meanings. Adults need to use clear and simple language with toddlers. Instead of offering a lengthy and detailed rationale for why it's time for bed, parents will find it more effective to say, for example, "It's time to get ready for bed now," and initiate one at a time each element of the bedtime routine: "Now let's (pick and say one at a time) have our snack ... take our bath ... read our story" and so forth.

- *Offer choices.* Toddlers exert their sense of autonomy by using the magic word "No!" Caregivers should not ask, "Do you want to take your nap now?" when desiring an affirmative answer. Instead, they can ask, "Which of these books do you want to read before nap time?" At mealtime, they can ask, "Would you like juice or milk with your lunch?" The key is to offer (only) two acceptable choices, and then let the child make the decision.

- *Set limits.* Toddlers will push the limits until they find the boundaries that keep them feeling safe. When adults provide no boundaries, children often become anxious and ill-tempered from the resulting insecurity. Adults can say simply to a child, "I will not let you hurt the baby," "I know you're angry, but you cannot call me names," or "We don't throw our food." When setting limits, caregivers will need to assist children in complying by using other strategies described in this section.

• *Use forecasting.* As mentioned above, very young children do not have the sense of time and life experience to know what will happen tomorrow or even in the next hour. They're often rudely surprised and behave accordingly when caregivers swoop them off to their child care center on Monday morning after a pleasant weekend at home. When parents say to a child at bedtime, "Tomorrow, we get to [not 'have to'] go to . . . [Carol's house, school, etc.]," they are giving him or her the knowledge of what is coming next. They remind him or her again in the morning when they wake the child up: "Today, we get to go to. . . . " Informed children feel more mastery and control and are often less resistant. A more immediate and equally useful version of forecasting is giving 5- and 2-minute warnings (no stop watch is required—remember, children have an undeveloped sense of time): "In 5 minutes, we need to go home. . . . In 2 minutes, we'll go home. . . . It's time to go; let's get our coats on."

• *Offer daily opportunities for physical activity.* This may seem obvious, but in our sedentary television culture, many children do not get the exercise and physical activity they require for a healthy body and reasonably cheerful disposition. Outdoor play areas are best if they are safe and accessible. However, even in confined indoor spaces, caregivers can create obstacle courses of pillows and chairs for children to crawl over and under. Parents or caregivers can play chase with children, sail and retrieve paper airplanes, roll a ball back and forth, or ask toddlers to walk their baby dolls in their doll strollers. Resources in our bibliography offer multiple ideas for infant and toddler activities for both indoors and outdoors, many of which involve movement.

• *Limit and monitor television and video watching.* The American Academy of Pediatrics recommends no more than 1 or 2 hours of television or video watching per day for young children. Most importantly, anything more restricts the time children need to interact with and explore their world. Additionally, commercial television creates appetites for sugary and fat-filled foods and for toys that are often not conducive to learning and creative play. Finally, it's important to ensure that young children do not view programs (these can include television news, Internet sites, or CD-ROMs) that have violence, explicit sex, or other content that will be confusing and potentially frightening for them.

• *Use redirection and substitution.* When toddlers are playing with objects adults don't want them to have or pounding on surfaces they may damage, instead of yelling "No!," caregivers can remove the offending object and hand them an acceptable one, or offer them a cooking pot to bang on instead the glass coffee table. In the kitchen, toddlers can reach unbreakable plastic containers if they are kept in a low cupboard. When parents or caregivers are busy at the stove or sink, children can be safely busy nearby, as they dump, sort, and stack the plastic ware. Dog obedience trainers stress that just using the word "No" with a dog is not useful, because it does not tell the dog what we want it to do. It only suggests immediate cessation of activity. The same is true when using this word with children. Giving, telling, or showing children an acceptable alternative to an unacceptable or undesirable behavior will be much more productive.

SUMMARY

It is in parenting behaviors that "the rubber meets the road," so to speak. A parent's wishes, hopes, and good intentions are lost on a young child. Infants and toddlers know only what they experience through tasting, touching, hearing, or seeing. They experience their parents' love through actions: sensitivity to cries; respect for privacy when baby doesn't want to be tickled or fed; arrangement of the physical environment to allow for physical mobility and exploration; words that teach and soothe; and limits that protect, clarify, and guide.

But such behaviors are not always automatic, even when parents have the best intentions. And teaching those behaviors is not always straightforward. We turn next to those factors that underlie parenting behavior, beginning in the next chapter with beliefs and attitudes that can either support or hinder parents from effectively meeting the needs of their children.

REFERENCES

Ainsworth, M. D. S., Blehar, M. C., Waters, E., & Wall, S. (1978). *Patterns of attachment: A psychological study of the Strange Situation.* Hillsdale, NJ: Erlbaum.

Arend, R., Gove, F., & Sroufe, L. A. (1979). Continuity of individual adaption from infancy to kindergarten: A predictive study of ego-resiliency and curiosity in preschoolers. *Child Development, 50, 950–959.*

Bakermans-Kranenburg, M. J., & Juffer, F. (1996, July). *Putting the train on a different track.* Symposium presented to the World Association of Infant Mental Health, Tampere, Finland.

Barnard, K. E. (1979). *Instructor's learning resource manual.* Seattle: NCAST Publications, University of Washington.

Beckwith, L., Cohen, S. E., Kopp, C. B., Parmelee, A. H., & Marcy, T. G. (1976). Caregiver–infant interaction and early cognitive development in preterm infants. *Child Development, 47,* 579–587.

Begley, S. (1996, February 19). Your child's brain. *Newsweek, 127,* 55–58.

Belsky, J., & Nezworski, T. (Eds.). (1988). *Clinical implications of attachment.* Hillsdale, NJ: Erlbaum.

Bowlby, J. (1973). *Attachment and loss: Vol. 2. Separation.* New York: Basic Books.

Bowlby, J. (1980). *Attachment and loss: Vol. 3. Loss, sadness, and depression.* New York: Basic Books.

Bowlby, J. (1982). *Attachment and loss: Vol. 1. Attachment* (2nd ed.). New York: Basic Books.

Bradley, R. H., & Caldwell, B. M. (1984). The relation of infants' home environment to achievement test performance in first grade: A follow-up study. *Child Development, 55,* 803–809.

Bretherton, I., & Water, E. (Eds.). (1985). Growing points of attachment theory and research. *Monographs of the Society for Research in Child Development, 50*(1–2, Serial No. 209).

Butler, D. (1980). *Babies need books.* New York: Atheneum.

Carlson, E. A. (1998). A prospective longitudinal study of attachment disorganization/disorientation. *Child Development, 69,* 1107–1128.

Cicchetti, D., & Barnett, D. (1991). Attachment organization in maltreated preschoolers. *Development and Psychopathology, 4,* 397–412.

Clarke-Stewart, K. A. (1973). Interactions between mothers and their young children. *Monographs of the Society for Research in Child Development, 38*(7–9, Serial No. 153).

Crittenden, P. M. (1988). Relationships at risk. In J. Belsky & T. Nezworski (Eds.), *Clinical implications of attachment* (pp. 136–174). Hillsdale, NJ: Erlbaum.

Dunst, C. J., & Trivette, C. M. (1990). Assessment of social support in early intervention programs. In S. J. Meisels & J. P. Shonkoff (Eds.), *Handbook of early childhood intervention* (pp. 326–349). New York: Cambridge University Press.

Egeland, B., & Erickson, M. F. (1987). Psychologically unavailable caregiving. In M. R. Brassard, R. Germain, & S. N. Hart (Eds.), *Psychological maltreatment of children and youth* (pp. 110–120). New York: Pergamon Press.

Egeland, B., & Erickson, M. F. (1990). Rising above the past: Strategies for helping new mothers break the cycle of abuse and neglect. *Zero to Three, 11,* 29–35.

Egeland, B., & Farber, E. A. (1984). Infant–mother attachment: Factors related to its development and changes over time. *Child Development, 55,* 753–771.

Epstein, A. S. (1980). *Assessing the child development information needed by adolescent parents with very young children.* Ypsilanti, MI: High/Scope Educational Research Foundation. (ERIC Document Reproduction Service No. ED 183 286)

Erickson, M. F. (1984). *Developmental antecedents of individual differences in compliance in young children.* Unpublished doctoral dissertation, University of Minnesota, Minneapolis.

Erickson, M. F. (1989). The STEEP program: Helping young families rise above "at-risk." *Family Resource Coalition Report, 8,* 14–15.

Erickson, M. F. (1999). *Seeing is believing: A training videotape.* Minneapolis: University of Minnesota.

Erickson, M. F., & Egeland, B. (1987). A developmental view of the psychological consequences of maltreatment. *School Psychology Review, 16,* 156–168.

Erickson, M. F., & Egeland, B. (1996). Child neglect. In J. Briere, L. Berliner, J. Bulkley, C. Jenny, & T. Reid (Eds.), *The APSAC handbook on child maltreatment* (pp. 4–20). Thousand Oaks, CA: Sage.

Erickson, M. F., Egeland, B., & Pianta, R. (1989). The effects of maltreatment on the development of young children. In D. Cicchetti & V. Carlson (Eds.), *Child maltreatment* (pp. 647–684). New York: Cambridge University Press.

Erickson, M. F., Korfmacher, J., & Egeland, B. (1992). Attachments past and present: Implications for therapeutic intervention with mother–infant dyads. *Development and Psychopathology, 4,* 495–507.

Erickson, M. F., & Pianta, R. C. (1985, April). *Behavior problems in young children: Early identification and prevention.* Paper presented at the annual meeting of the National Association of School Psychologists, Philadelphia.

Erickson, M. F., & Pianta, R. C. (1989). New lunchbox, old feelings: What kids bring to school. *Early Education and Development, 1,* 35–49.

Erickson, M. F., Sroufe, L. A., & Egeland, B. (1985). The relationship between quality of attachment and behavior problems in preschool in a high-risk sample. In I. Bretherton & E. Waters (Eds.), Growing points of attachment theory and research. *Monographs of the Society for Research in Child Development, 50*(1–2, Serial No. 209), 147–166.

Erikson, E. (1963). *Childhood and society* (2nd ed.). New York: Norton.

Goodman, Y. (1986). Children coming to know literacy. In W. Teale & E. Sulzby (Eds.), *Emergent literacy: Writing and reading* (pp. 1–14). Norwood, NJ: Ablex.

Greenberg, M., Cicchetti, D., & Cummings, E. M. (Eds.). (1990). *Attachment in the preschool years: Theory, research, and intervention.* Chicago: University of Chicago Press.

Greenough, W., Black, J., & Wallace, C. (1987). Experience and brain development. *Child Development, 58,* 555–567.

Hart, B., & Risley, T. R. (1995). *Meaningful differences in the everyday experience of young American children.* Baltimore: Brookes.

Jalongo, M. R. (1990). *Early childhood language arts.* Boston: Allyn & Bacon.

Kennell, J. H., & Klaus, M. H. (Eds.). (1976). *Maternal infant bonding.* St. Louis: Mosby.

Kupetz, B. N., & Green, E. J. (1997). Sharing books with infants and toddlers: Facing the challenges. *Young Children, 52,* 22–27.

Lewis, M., Feiring, C., McGuffog, C., & Jaskir, J. (1984). Predicting psychopathology in 6-year-olds from early social relations. *Child Development, 55,* 123–136.

MacTurk, R. H., McCarthy, M. E., Vietze, P. M., & Yarrow, L. J. (1987). Sequential analysis of mastery behavior in 6- and 12-month old infants. *Developmental Psychology, 23*, 199–203.

MacTurk, R. H., Vietze, P. M., McCarthy, M. E., McQuiston, S., & Yarrow, L. J. (1985). The organization of exploratory behavior in Down syndrome and nondelayed infants. *Child Development, 56*, 573–581.

Main, M., & Hesse, E. (1990). Parents' unresolved traumatic experiences are related to infant disorganized attachment status: Is frightened and/or frightening parental behavior the linking mechanism? In M. T. Greenberg, D. Cicchetti, & E. M. Cummings (Eds.), *Attachment in the preschool years* (pp. 161–182). Chicago: University of Chicago Press.

Main, M., & Solomon, J. (1990). Procedures for identifying infants as disorganized/disoriented during the Ainsworth Strange Situation. In M. T. Greenberg, D. Cicchetti, & E. M. Cummings (Eds.), *Attachment in the preschool years* (pp. 121–160). Chicago: University of Chicago Press.

Nash, J. M. (1997, February 3). Fertile minds. *Time, 149*, 48–56.

Nugent, K. J. (1985). *Using the NBAS with infants and their families: Guidelines for intervention.* New York: March of Dimes.

Ogawa, J. R., Sroufe, L. A., Weinfield, N. S., Carlson, E., & Egeland, B. (1997). Development and the fragmented self: A longitudinal study of dissociative symptomatology in a nonclinical sample. *Development and Psychopathology, 4*, 855–879.

Osofsky, H. J., & Osofsky, J. D. (1970). Adolescents as mothers: Results of a program for low-income pregnant teenagers with some emphasis upon infants' development. *American Journal of Orthopsychiatry, 40*, 825–834.

Piaget, J. (1952). *The origins of intelligence in children.* New York: International Universities Press.

Ramey, C. T., & Ramey, S. L. (1992). Effective early intervention. *Mental Retardation, 30*, 337–435.

Rode, S. S., Chang, P. N., Fisch, R. O., & Sroufe, L. A. (1981). Attachment patterns of infants separated at birth. *Developmental Psychology, 17*, 188–191.

Shore, R. (1997). *Rethinking the brain: New insights into early development.* New York: Families and Work Institute.

Singer, L. M., Brodzinsky, D. M., Ramsay, D., Stein, M., & Waters, E. (1985). Mother–infant attachment in adoptive families. *Child Development, 56*, 1543–1551.

Sroufe, L. A. (1983). Infant–caregiver attachment and patterns of adaptation in preschool: The roots of maladaptation and competence. In M. Perlmutter (Ed.), *Minnesota Symposia in Child Psychology. Vol. 16. Development and policy concerning children with special needs* (pp. 41–83). Hillsdale, NJ: Erlbaum.

Sumner, G., & Spietz, A. (1994). *NCAST caregiver/parent–child interaction feeding manual.* Seattle: NCAST Publications, University of Washington, School of Nursing.

Taylor, D. (1983). *Family literacy: Young children learning to read and write.* Portsmouth, NH: Heinemann.

Thoman, E., & Browder, S. (1987). *Born dancing: How intuitive parents understand their baby's unspoken language and natural rhythms.* New York: Harper & Row.

Williamson, G. G. (1988, March). Motor control as a resource for adaptive coping. *Zero to Three, 9,* 1–7.

Yarrow, L. J., Rubenstein, J. L., & Pederson, F. A. (1975). *Infant and environment: Early cognitive and motivational development.* New York: Wiley.

FOUR

Enhancing Parental Knowledge and Understanding

Every time my husband or I step out of Jason's sight, he starts crying and comes crawling to look for us. He is so clingy, I just don't know how he'll ever survive in this world! When he was a tiny baby, we always went to him when he cried. Everyone told us we'd spoil him rotten, and I guess they were right.
　　　　　　　　　—DAWN, Mother of an 8-month-old

Dawn's concern about her baby's clinginess is not unusual. But, as you know, her baby's behavior is not unusual either. At 8 months old, Jason's need to keep his parents in sight is his way of saying that they are the most important people in his life right now, his source of security—just as they should be. As he matures and learns through experience that his parents will always come back for him, he will be able to tolerate longer and more frequent separations, carrying within himself the security they have given him.

Dawn's statement reflects the popular spoiling myth and a relatively common misunderstanding about the meaning of a child's separation anxiety. It will be to the advantage of both Jason and his family if these parents can recognize how normal their son's behavior is, what his separation protest means in the context of his developmental stage, and what they can do to provide a sense of security for him through this period despite possible criticism from friends and family members.

Supporting parents such as Dawn and her husband as they build their knowledge and understanding of their child's behavior is a central function of early intervention. This is not simply a matter of giving parents information, as if we had the answers and they did not. Rather it is a matter of joining with parents in an examination of what they believe, supporting them as they question and challenge those beliefs, and encouraging them to gather information from a variety of sources so that they can make informed choices about what will be best for them and their child.

In this chapter, we present a framework for enhancing parental understanding as a way to strengthen the parent–child relationship and promote the child's optimal development. Specifically, we consider how some crucial aspects of parental knowledge and understanding of child development influence parenting behavior; discuss parental awareness and understanding as constructs that change developmentally over the course of a parent's life and experience; examine some of the factors that support or interfere with parents' application of what they know; and present some strategies that we have found useful in working with parents to expand and deepen their understanding of their child's development and their relationship with their child.

KNOWLEDGE OF EARLY BEHAVIOR
AND DEVELOPMENT

To a large extent, parental behavior is a function of what parents know and understand about children's development and capabilities at different ages and stages. Knowledge informs the beliefs parents hold about child rearing and the expectations they have for their child's behavior. In working with families and infants, one of the first aspects of parental knowledge we encounter is recognition of the capabilities of the infant. Because a newborn baby is unable to speak or move around the room and is dependent on adults for his or her very survival, it is easy to overlook the remarkable competencies that the baby does possess. Adults sometimes seem to view the newborn as a little doll, rather than an already complex human being with a broad range of feelings and capabilities.

For many years, even physicians and child development professionals grossly underestimated the abilities of infants. For example, until not long ago parents were told that newborns are unable to see. Yet in the 1980s, research demonstrated that very young babies can recognize their parents by sight and sound (Nugent, 1985). When various adults are in the room, the infant consistently will turn toward the familiar face or voice of the parent. Other research has shown that within a few hours after birth, a baby will imitate the facial expression of an adult.

Meltzoff's (Meltzoff & Moore, 1983) groundbreaking photographs of tiny babies using their mouths and eyes to mimic the researcher's face can be quite amazing to those of us who grew up thinking of newborns as passive little creatures who barely know what is happening around them!

Some of the new findings regarding infants' sensitivities and capabilities can be alarming. For example, the research of Megan Gunnar and her associates has challenged long-held beliefs about newborns' insensitivity to pain (Gunnar, Malone, & Fisch, 1985). Contrary to popular beliefs and medical practices, newborns do experience the pain of circumcision, needle pricks, and other invasive medical procedures. As a result of this research, many clinics and hospitals are modifying their practices with infants. And parents certainly should take this new information into account as they make medical decisions involving their newborn children.

Nugent (1985) has developed a useful guide for professionals to use to help parents discover their newborn infant's capabilities (see annotated resource bibliography at the end of this book). Based on the work of Brazelton and his Neonatal Behavioral Assessment Scale (Brazelton, 1973), Nugent's brief intervention strategy has been shown to promote more positive interaction between parent and baby.

When parents confront the birth of a child with a disability, there is a special need for supportive intervention. More effective diagnostic techniques have made it more common for a disability to be identified at or shortly after birth. Cardone and Gilkerson (1992) describe their successful use of Family Administered Neonatal Activities, a short-term intervention program based on the Brazelton (1973) scale, which they have adapted specifically to parents whose babies are diagnosed with Down syndrome. Beginning as soon as a tentative diagnosis has been presented to the parents, this intervention helps parents begin to look past the disability to focus on the child as a human being with capabilities. Of course this short-term intervention is only the beginning; the birth of a child with a disability typically signals the loss of the dream of a normal child, and, as discussed later, grieving and adjustment are a long process.

In our own work, videotaping is one of the best tools we have found for expanding parents' knowledge of their newborn's capabilities. As described in Chapter 3, videotaping parents and babies allows the parents and professionals to discover together what the baby can do. This is especially helpful with babies whose disabilities may tend to obscure their competencies. For example, it is amazing to watch even tiny babies begin to use sound to compensate for their lack of sight as they get to know their mothers and fathers.

Knowledge of Developmental Sequences

A related issue for intervention is parental knowledge of normal developmental sequences, knowledge that helps to determine the behavioral expectations that parents have for their children as they mature. Whereas adults may tend to *under*estimate the capabilities of a newborn, they often *over*estimate the capabilities of children as they get older, and expect cooperation and self-control that are not realistic at that stage of the child's development. For example, parents may expect their children to sit still and entertain themselves for extended periods of time, long before children normally are capable of such sustained attention and independence. Of course as parents, most of us have longed for the chance to finish household chores or make a phone call while our children occupy themselves quietly. But when parents expect more than children are capable of delivering, there are negative results for both parent and child. See Table 4.1 for infant/toddler behaviors that are commonly the focus of inappropriate expectations by parents and caregivers.

Realistically, except when they're sleeping, infants and toddlers require almost constant vigilance and guidance in order to keep themselves and the world around them safe, not to mention happy. For parents, understanding this is the starting point for finding new ways to balance child rearing and the other demands on their time and energy. Parents will still feel frustrated that their time is so seldom their own, but

TABLE 4.1. Inappropriate Expectations for Infants and Toddlers

Sleeping through the night

Holding the bottle independently

Following an adult-driven feeding schedule

Regulating feelings and emotions

Understanding the meaning of the word "no"

Being ready for toilet training (and staying dry through the night)

Having the motor control to prevent rough, clumsy behavior

Understanding cause and effect (particularly with regard to own behavior)

Paying attention for an extended period of time

Remembering lessons from day to day or week to week

Generalizing a rule from one setting to another

Developing a taste for grown-up foods (babies experience sour or bitter tastes
   more intensely than adults do)

Putting toys away independently

Remaining quiet in settings such as movie theaters or church this is less likely to turn into intense anger if they have accurate knowledge about children's capabilities and needs.

Sometimes we adults get fooled into thinking children understand more than they actually do. For example, we often hear parents say something like, "I don't know why she is playing with the knobs on that TV. We just went through this the other day at home, and I taught her not to do that." Even young toddlers can learn to inhibit behavior if they are firmly told "No," and directed toward something else. But after a couple of days, they may forget. Or, as is often the case, they may not generalize the rule to a new setting. The parent may really believe that the child "knows better" than to play with the knobs on the TV. But the child may not be mature enough to remember that rule over a period of several days or to know that the rule applies to all TVs and not just the one on which he or she learned. Long-term memory and the ability to generalize learning from one situation to another are not yet developed in toddlers.

Sometimes a baby's eagerness to explore gets him or her into trouble. For example, at a recent parent education session, four babies aged 9–12 months were playing on the floor. Brian, with a big smile on his face, reached over to pat Christine's face. The pats were pretty vigorous and landed right in Christine's eye! As Christine started to cry, Brian's mother grabbed him and shouted, "Stop that! Don't be so mean!" You've probably seen similar situations with the parents and babies you know. How would you respond to Brian's mother? What do you think would be helpful for her to know about what Brian is capable of doing and understanding at 10 months of age?

We find that parents sometimes do not understand the following:

- Babies learn by exploring with their hands, by touching, grabbing, patting, even pinching or pulling.
- Babies lack both the motor control and the impulse control to touch in a way that is smooth and gentle.
- Babies are not cognitively mature enough to understand that it hurts others when they touch them roughly.

Brian is not old enough to learn the no-hitting rule, but he is old enough for his parents to take his hand, help him pat Christine softly, and say, "Be gentle." Over time, he will learn what is acceptable behavior, as he develops the physical and emotional ability to control his own actions.

What is most important in this kind of situation is to help parents understand that the child is not just willfully being "bad," but really is not mature enough to live up to the parents' expectations. Of course, there are times when children *are* being willfully noncompliant. See

Chapter 3 for a discussion of limit setting and behavior guidance for very young children.

ENCOURAGING PARENTS
TO SUSTAIN THEIR OWN LEARNING

There are many fine sources of information about child development and the behaviors parents realistically can expect of children in the early months and years of life. A wide variety of useful supports are listed in the resource section at the end of this book. Introducing parents to these resources is ultimately far more effective than setting ourselves up as the "experts." With access to multiple resources, parents build on their own expertise and develop the confidence to match.

Although child development books are helpful to parents whose children are developing within normal expectations, parents of children with special needs often have less to guide them. Rates of development may be highly variable among children and even across domains of development for any individual child. (For example, motor behavior may be normal or advanced while language behavior is significantly delayed.) And for some children, their behaviors may be idiosyncratic and unlike any other child, even one with a similar diagnosis. As described in detail in Chapter 3, videotaping can be a wonderful tool to help parents focus on their child's unique capabilities and his or her own developmental timetable. Parents and professionals can experiment together, "testing the limits" of what a child can do. Capturing that experience on video allows for careful analysis afterwards, as well as monitoring changes in the child's behavior and abilities over time.

> *Three-year-old David was confined to a wheelchair, had frequent and severe seizures, and was believed to have almost no voluntary muscle control. Sometimes he appeared to reach out with his arm as if to touch something, but his parents and doctors couldn't tell for sure if the movement was deliberate or random. David spoke no words, and his parents were uncertain whether he understood them when they spoke.*
>
> *But David did have a beautiful smile that lit up his face when his parents looked into his eyes, and he could turn his head to seek their gaze. David's expressive face also gave a clear indication of what his favorite—and least favorite—foods were. With that in mind, his parents decided to test the limits of his verbal understanding by asking him to show them with his eyes what treat he would like. After repeated trials and coaching, David soon was responding easily to his parents' mealtime question, "What do you want to eat?" With a smile and a steady gaze he would "point" with his eyes*

to the item on the table that caught his fancy. Soon, his parents were using the same strategy to let him make age-appropriate choices as to which shirt to wear or which book he wanted them to read to him.

For all parents, and perhaps especially for parents of children with disabilities, it is critical that they have opportunities to see other children in similar circumstances and be with other parents who face comparable challenges (see Chapter 5 for a discussion of parent support groups). A variety of child and family advocacy groups and resource centers are eager to help parents learn more about what they can expect as their special needs child develops. Several of these are listed in the resource section at the end of this book.

Understanding the Developmental Meaning of Child Behavior

Even more important than knowledge of developmental sequences and timetables is understanding the developmental meaning of a child's behavior. The misunderstanding of behavior can lead to the attribution of negative characteristics to either the child or the parents (Egeland & Breitenbucher, 1980; Newberger & Cook, 1983; Sameroff & Feil, 1985), as in the case of two frequently misinterpreted behaviors discussed below.

The first is separation anxiety, which usually appears by 7–8 months of age and may last well into the toddler period. As illustrated in the vignette about Dawn and Jason at the beginning of this chapter, sometimes parents take separation protest as a sign that the baby is spoiled, demanding, inappropriately dependent, and overly fussy. And/or they may feel that they are bad parents to have created such a difficult child. Many parents worry from the first days of the child's life that they will spoil their baby by responding consistently to his or her cries, so separation protests confirm their worst fears. Relief and reassurance come with the understanding that separation protest is a normal, healthy phenomenon that indicates that the baby now recognizes that the caregiver still exists even when out of sight (Piaget's notion of object permanence, 1952); that the caregiver has appropriately become important as a source of security for the child; and that as the child's needs for closeness continue to be satisfied, he or she gradually will become more able to separate and increasingly independent (Ainsworth, Blehar, Waters, & Wall, 1978; Erickson, Sroufe, & Egeland, 1985; Sroufe, Fox, & Pancake, 1983).

A second commonly misunderstood behavior is toddler negativism, which parents again may take as a sign that the child is "nasty" or "spoiled" or "just like Uncle George"—or, alternatively, as a sign that they have failed as parents by allowing this little monster to go unleashed. It is liberating for parents to understand that the toddler's negativism is the tool that the child uses to begin to establish a separate sense of self and to exercise newfound autonomy, which are major developmental accomplishments. As discussed in Chapter 3, toddlers need clear, consistent limits to protect them from an overwhelming sense of chaos. They also need opportunities to make choices and act independently within those limits (see Breger, 1974, for an excellent discussion of this developmental period).

When child behaviors trigger negative attributions, one way to intervene is to "reframe" the behaviors verbally for parents, reinterpreting the behavior as reflecting a positive motive or characteristic in the child. (This is not to dismiss how upsetting or exhausting the behaviors can be for parents, but just to balance the picture with a different point of view.) Table 4.2 presents a brief list of behaviors that often trigger negative attributions, followed by ways they can be positively reframed for parents.

Practicing Perspective Taking

Reframing behavior is one step toward perspective taking, helping parents to see the situation in a fresh way, through the eyes of the child. Perspective taking is a key component of good relationships in general, and an invaluable tool for parents and others who care for young children. Following are several strategies aimed at supporting parents' in looking at things from the child's point of view.

TALKING FOR THE BABY

This is a simple, informal strategy that can be used easily during home visits, group sessions with parents and babies, or even during a quick chat when a parent is picking a baby up from child care. For example, if we see a baby pushing the bottle away as the mother insists on feeding her, we may say in a small voice, "Hey, Mom, I've had enough for now." Or, when a toddler is cranky and clingy during our visit, we might voice his feelings by saying, "It sure is hard for me to share your attention for such a long time." One colleague told us that after several months of speaking for the babies, she noticed parents doing the same with each other's babies, a good sign that they were in a perspective-taking frame of mind.

A similar strategy can be used in a more structured way. For example, Osofsky and her colleagues (Carter, Osofsky, & Hann, 1991) sys-

TABLE 4.2. Reframing Infant Behavior

Behavior	Negative attribution	Reframe
Crying	She's just trying to get at me.	She sure lets you know when she needs something.
	She's such a brat.	She's really able to tell you what she wants.
Thumb sucking	He's such a wimp. He's going to ruin his teeth.	Isn't it great that he's found a way to comfort himself?
Separation protest	She's so spoiled. I can't move without her hanging on my leg.	You sure are special to her. She really knows you'll take care of her.
Getting into things and making messes	What a pain in the neck! He won't ever stay out of my stuff.	He's so curious and eager to learn. He wants to see and touch everything. That must be exciting for him.
Saying "no!"	She's so defiant. She'd better learn some respect fast!	She's becoming so strong and independent. She needs to show you she has a mind of her own.

Note. From Christenson and Conoley (1992). Copyright 1992 by the National Association of School Psychologists. Reprinted by permission of the publisher.

tematically ask young mothers to use first-person language to say what they think their baby is feeling and communicating with his or her expressions and body language. These clinician/researchers also encourage the young mothers to take turns speaking for each other's babies, giving them further practice in perspective taking.

LETTERS FROM THE BABY

A more formal extension of talking for the baby, letters written to parents in the voice of the child have proven to be an especially powerful tool for promoting perspective taking. Speaking to those most important attachment issues, one letter from an 8-month-old who always wanted Mom in sight said, "You are the most important thing in my life right now. . . . I'd crawl for miles on my hands and knees just to see your face. . . . Sometimes even just hearing your voice is enough to make me feel okay." While we often write letters that address normative developmental issues (see sample letter about the importance of talking to babies in Chapter 3, Table 3.4), we also sometimes tailor a letter to an individual family's particular issues. This is especially helpful when a child has special needs or a parent has a unique, "hot button" response to a particular issue.

Parents have told us that these letters touch them emotionally and often cast their child's behavior in a new light, enabling them to move out of a dead-end pattern in dealing with troublesome behaviors. For example, one mother said she was getting locked in repeated power struggles with her son when it was time to put his toys away, but when she read one of our letters on that topic, it woke her up to what her son needed.

A variation on this strategy, appropriate for parents who are comfortable with written activities, is to ask the parents to write a letter as if it is from their child. If parents are willing to share what they write, this can provide a great starting point for a one-to-one or group discussion.

PHYSICAL EXERCISES IN PERSPECTIVE TAKING

Although many intervention strategies are primarily verbal, sometimes a physical experience is worth a thousand words. For example, in one parent group session, several mothers were seated around a table with one arm stretched in the air. At the direction of their facilitator, they sat this way for several minutes, eventually squirming and groaning about how uncomfortable they were. What was the point? Well, these mothers had toddlers who were often resistant to holding Mom's hand when they were walking in a public place. Of course, for safety reasons the mothers were right in insisting that the children hold on, but some of the mothers were getting really angry about the fuss their kids were making. This little exercise was designed to help them see from the child's point of view how uncomfortable it can be to reach up and hold hands. On another occasion, a group of teen mothers of young infants had been complaining about their babies' crying every time they wanted something. The group facilitator placed a plate of freshly baked cookies on the table and asked the young women to pretend that they could not speak or reach the cookies: "How does it feel to see and smell something that you want, but not know how to go about getting it?"

VIDEOTAPING TO ENCOURAGE PERSPECTIVE TAKING

The use of videotaping, as described earlier, is another powerful way of helping parents see through the eyes of the child. When we watch the tapes with parents, we question and comment in a way that invites the parents to discover what the baby is experiencing and communicating. For example, we might say, "Look at that expression on his face. I wonder what he was feeling then." Or we might observe, "That must be quite a shock to feel that bath water for the first time when you're too little to know what to expect."

CHILDHOOD MEMORIES AS A PATHWAY TO PERSPECTIVE TAKING

One tool that we all have to help us gain perspective with children is our own memory. Although memories are shaped and modified by our adult knowledge and experience, it can be very helpful to dig back into our childhood as we try to understand what is going on with our children now. Do you remember, for example, a relative who was overbearing with hugs and kisses? How did you feel when your parents insisted that you go to bed when you wanted nothing more than to snuggle up with them on the couch?

USING MUSIC, POETRY, FICTION, AND QUOTATIONS TO ENCOURAGE PERSPECTIVE TAKING

In this simple group activity, we listen to a relevant song or read aloud a passage from poetry, fiction, or biography that addresses an issue of interest to the group. For example, we might read a passage from a current novel about domestic violence or parent–child relationships. Then we talk together about the feelings elicited, themes expressed, underlying assumptions and values of the characters, and how our own life experiences have been similar or different. As with all of our activities, we look for opportunities to tie the discussion to the experience of young children, supporting the parents' abilities to see through their children's eyes. Another example, with a focus on how children develop self-esteem, is to listen to a recording of the Whitney Houston song "The Greatest Love of All." Then guided by open-ended questioning, parents discuss the meaning of the song, whether it is essential to love oneself before loving others, how one learns to love oneself, and, most importantly, what this means for parents and their children.

Perspective taking reflects a relatively high level of parental awareness and understanding. Some researchers have proposed a developmental framework for how parental understanding progresses with maturation, learning, and experience, moving from totally egocentric views (i.e., seeing only the parent's needs) to a much more sophisticated way of understanding children's points of view, their changing developmental parameters, and varied contexts in which behavior occurs (Newberger, 1980; Newberger & Cook, 1983; Sameroff & Feil, 1985). However, research has yielded few suggestions on how to help parents systematically progress from one level of understanding to the next. Furthermore, although a certain level of understanding seems to be a prerequisite for sensitive parenting behavior, it does not necessarily follow that changing parental understanding will automatically produce a change in parenting behavior. This is an area that is still ripe for research.

Encountering Parental Resistance to New Learning

Many parents are highly motivated to learn all that they can about their child's behavior and development. However, for many reasons, some parents are resistant to developing new insight. For example, a teen mother might believe she knows all there is to know and that no adult, including the most well-meaning parent educator, could possibly know anything that would speak to her experience. This attitude reflects common adolescent developmental issues (i.e., the need to do it "my way," to learn from "my own" mistakes), but also may be intensified by the kind of life history that is common among teenagers who become parents. Children whose own attachment and autonomy issues have not been well resolved are most likely to become teen parents. So, much like toddlers who are fighting valiantly for their own autonomy, these teen parents may scorn the experience and wisdom of well-meaning adults. Of course turning 20 does not instantly make such resistance disappear. For a variety of reasons, older parents may also be resistant to new learning.

Research on the effectiveness of intervention has not yet yielded much in the way of specific strategies that overcome parental resistance. But our own experience with young parents, as well as the wisdom of other professionals that has informed our work, suggests several ways to encourage resistant parents to be more open to new learning.

First of all, we begin by attending to the parent's own feelings. We listen carefully and attentively to his or her needs and concerns rather than jumping right away to a focus on the child's needs. Then we frame our discussion in terms of what will help this parent accomplish his or her own goals. For example, it may be in a mother's interest to get the child to bed at a reasonable time so that she can have time to study or watch a favorite TV show. Although we might wish that the mother would focus more on the child's needs, by meeting her where she is, we will be more likely to help her move forward.

When we encounter a parent who is totally invested in a belief that we are certain is wrong, it is very tempting to throw up our arms and say, "I can't believe you think like that!" But head-on confrontation is rarely effective. Particularly with adolescents, confrontation and argument often only intensify people's commitment to their own points of view. Giving parents a way to expand their thinking without losing face is ultimately much more effective. Instead of direct confrontation, we might say, "That's one way to think about it. Another way might be. . . . "

We have found that we may not see the effect of this strategy right away, but perhaps later parents will have claimed this new perspective as their own. For example, one young mother was convinced that she was going to spoil her baby if she got up with her in the night. We acknowledged that many people thought that way, then gently nudged her to consider a different point of view. A few weeks later, she told her group that she had discovered that it was much better to respond to her baby's cries. (We carefully avoided saying, "I told you so.")

Sometimes young parents are more open to teaching when it comes from a peer rather than someone with a generational age difference. In a group setting, it often is helpful to find a peer who is on the right track and to support that person in being the "teacher" to the others. The risk in this is that it can set up a kind of "sibling rivalry" among group members if it looks like we're playing favorites, so this strategy needs to be used carefully and with a focus on finding what each member has to offer to the others.

By being a careful listener, we often can find ways to link the parenting message we want to convey to the parents' own observations. For example, one mother was invested in physical punishment, convinced that spanking was necessary to teach her child "who was in charge." But this same mother also observed, "No matter how hard I spank her, she still keeps throwing those tantrums at bedtime." In that case, we could say, "You've discovered that spanking isn't working. I wonder what other ideas you have about what might work." From that, we can engage the parent in speculating about what the child is experiencing and brainstorming about more effective ways to help the child settle down.

Finally, it is effective to support the parent in being an investigator, affirming his or her ability to figure things out. For example, in the case described above, a next step would be to support the mother in trying a new approach for a week or two, carefully keeping track of the child's response. With encouragement, she might figure out that the child needs some quiet time and some special attention from Mom right before bedtime. She may need to start this routine an hour earlier than she usually does in order to meet her own goals. She might even be interested in keeping a simple chart of her progress and then later share her findings with other parents in the group. This approach takes into account her own need for private time in the evening, as well as the child's needs for a comforting bedtime routine. And it affirms that she is the ultimate "expert" on her own child.

Factors That Mitigate Day-to-Day Application of Parental Knowledge

Knowing and understanding child development and behavior is one thing; using that knowledge in daily life with children is sometimes quite another matter. There are many factors that influence how people apply their parenting knowledge, some having to do with the inner life of the parent and others having to do with life circumstances, stressors, and available support. We discuss some of these external factors in more detail in Chapter 5, but summarize them here as a reminder that early intervention is not only about helping parents learn what children need, but about working with parents to overcome some of the barriers that may interfere with their ability to carry through on what they know is best. As with so much of what we have discussed in this book, this is a universal issue. In our own lives as parents, we are constantly confronted with the fact that despite advanced degrees in child development, our behavior as parents reflects our emotional status and a whole range of life experiences, both positive and negative. To work with parents around daily application of parental knowledge means sharing the journey with them as the vulnerable and complex people that we all are.

One of the most crucial factors accounting for how parents apply their knowledge is the degree to which the parents are supported by others. This begins with day-to-day support in the home, in the form of shared parenting and mutual emotional support between two adults who both love the child. Today many parents struggle on their own without that basic in-home support, and many do a valiant job in spite of the fact that they do not have someone with whom to share the daily joys and challenges of parenting. Whether parents are single or have a partner, they do best when they have other sources of support from extended family, friends, and both informal and formal resources in their community. In all of our lives, there is a delicate balance between stress and support. When our daily stress exceeds our available support, our best knowledge sometimes flies out the window. (In Chapter 5, we discuss in more detail research on the importance of support and its role in early intervention.)

A parent's ability to apply knowledge of child development is also a function of his or her personal status and feelings of self-worth. For example, it is hard to balance work and family; but when a parent's work is interesting and satisfying, and imparts a sense of purpose and worth, the parent is more likely to be an effective, sensitive parent. On the other hand, parenting is more difficult for the adult who sees few options for becoming self-supporting, feels like a failure because of a lack of education, or is working in a situation where he or she is not respected and feels little control over the future. Child rearing demands enormous spirit and energy, grounded in personal strength and a healthy sense of self.

A parent's feelings and actions toward a child also reflect a complex set of perceptions and emotions having to do with the child's characteristics and often even the circumstances of the baby's conception and birth. For example, a mother who did not want to be pregnant may unknowingly blame the child for complicating the mother's life or tying her down. Or, conversely, young parents who unrealistically expect a new baby to fill the huge, empty hole in their lives may be overwhelmed with disappointment when the baby fails to live up to that expectation. Sometimes parents see in their child qualities that trigger unpleasant associations. Such was the case with Lisa, whose baby daughter bore a strong resemblance to her father, a man with whom Lisa had had a "one-night stand" and who subsequently became a "monster" in Lisa's description. Thus Lisa's home visitor focused on helping Lisa see all of the qualities that were unique to her daughter and to recognize that she could be a strong influence on how her daughter eventually would turn out. It took a good deal of time and effort for Lisa to begin to see her daughter as a person in her own right, rather than a reembodiment of the man she preferred to forget.

When the Child Has a Disability

During pregnancy, most parents fantasize about the baby they will have, how they will be together as a family, and how that child will grow up. And although nearly all parents worry on some level about complications that can undermine the health of the baby, the birth of a child with disabilities usually comes as an enormous shock. Whether the disability is visible and diagnosable at birth (or, with modern technology, even before), or whether it gradually becomes evident at some later period, it almost always is experienced by the parents as a major loss—the loss of a dream, the loss of the imagined child. Particularly poignant on this topic is Moses (1988), a psychologist who had worked with parents of children with disabilities for many years and then suddenly and surprisingly learned first hand what "lost dreams" meant when his own baby was diagnosed with a severe disability. Parents of children with disabilities often tell us how valuable the Moses videotapes are. As one mother said, "He told my story before I even knew that's what I was experiencing."

As we have discussed throughout this book, the early months of life are critical for the child's learning and emotional development, and, as we have indicated in earlier sections, children with disabilities are no exception. Although they may learn and develop at different rates and, depending on the nature of their disability, through different modes, the relationship principles we have discussed are clearly applicable. And yet when parents are grappling with shock and, in many cases, denial following the diagnosis of a disability, their ability to become fully engaged and responsive to their baby may be seriously undermined. This is where the role of family support and early intervention becomes especially critical.

In general terms, the task of a professional working with the family is usually twofold: supporting the parents through the normal cycles of grief that follow the diagnosis and, at the same time, working with the parents to understand and adapt to the child's special needs and strengths. The baby cannot wait, no matter how much the parents' grief may demand our attention. And yet the parents are unlikely to feel strong enough to attend to the baby unless they are getting the support they need as they work through their feelings.

Given the nature of the grieving process, and the turning inward that is an intrinsic part of it, it often feels overwhelming to parents to try to muster the emotional energy that a baby demands. Many parents report feeling consumed by guilt that they somehow caused the disability or that they don't feel the love they believe they should feel for the child. It is common for parents to sink into a serious depression and to have suicidal thoughts. As with any depression, parents may pull away from the people and activities that they ordinarily would enjoy; yet, isolation and inactivity feed the depression. Furthermore, relatives and friends often are uncomfortable about how to act around the family, so they may pull away as well. Thus it is especially critical to focus on helping the parents stay connected to their natural support network and to maintain some level of normal activity to counteract the tendency to withdraw.

As described throughout this book, appropriate parent–infant intervention strategies include those that aim to identify this baby's unique strengths and competencies, interpret and respond to his or her signals, see through the baby's eyes, and form realistic behavioral expectations. But all of those strategies will need to be undertaken in the context of the parents' special feelings surrounding the disability. As we work with parent and baby, it may be helpful to reflect back, or name, the parent's feelings as we see them. For example, as a parent works to engage a baby in face-to-face interaction, we might acknowledge, "I can see that it's frustrating not to get the response that you hoped for." When a parent can see only what the baby is *not* able to do, we can play an important role in helping to focus his or her attention on what the baby *can* do, no matter how small or insignificant the accomplishment appears. Because each child is different, this will involve an ongoing process of experimentation to figure out with the parent what works best with this particular child.

As we work with the family, it will be important to keep in mind that grieving the loss of the imagined child is not a finite process. It goes on throughout the life of the child and often is intensely reactivated when the parents see their baby's normal age-mates achieving new milestones. For example, when other children start to walk or talk or when they go off to preschool, or even college, the parents of a child with disabilities often will go deeply into the grieving process again. Early in the life of the child is the time to help the parents establish healthy patterns for dealing with that recurring grief. We can suggest resources and acknowledge parents' strength as they accept the cyclical nature of grief and deal positively with its various manifestations.

According to countless parents, the most effective strategy of all is to join in mutual support with other parents in similar circumstances. In two-parent families it seems to be especially important that both partners participate. Many families have described the different ways that men and women handle their emotions and the conflict that often ensues between husbands and wives who are at different places in the grieving process. As we gathered information for this book, we talked to parents who have been actively involved in support groups for more than 10 years. As one mother said, "It is the thing that kept me alive and my marriage intact."

Exploring the Past, Looking to the Future

As we consider the many factors that support or hinder parents in applying their best knowledge of child development and parenting, one of the most important is how they were parented in their own childhood. Notably, recent research suggests that perhaps even more important than how they actually were parented is how they have come to think about the way they were cared for. Research on intergenerational cycles of maltreatment points to healthy resolution of childhood issues as a factor in accounting for parents who care well for their children even though the parents were abused in their own childhood (Egeland, 1988; Erickson, Korfmacher & Egeland, 1992). Similarly, attachment researchers point to such resolution as an important predictor of quality of attachment between the parent and baby (Fonagy, Steele, & Steele, 1991; Posada, Waters, Crowell, & Lay, 1995; Ricks, 1985).

A summary of these different bodies of research, reinforced by wisdom from clinical practice, suggests that resolution includes several components: facing the pain of the past; acknowledging its lasting influence; recognizing that at least to some degree, a person can choose what to repeat from the past and what not to; and then mustering all available resources to make it possible to act on those choices. Barriers to such resolution include denial of painful experiences, dismissal (e.g., "Oh yeah, my dad abused me but that has nothing to do with who I am now!"), or preoccupation with distressing childhood experiences. In any of those scenarios, a parent's emotional energy is tied up in defending against the pain of the past, which leaves him or her fewer resources for responding to the needs of a baby.

The manual for the STEEP program (Erickson & Simon, 1999) describes activities to help parents face the past and look to the future, choosing what they want to carry forward as they care for their children. Here we summarize briefly some of the strategies that have been especially effective. As we continue to explore ways to share this important journey with parents, we owe tribute to the pioneering infant mental health work of Fraiberg (1987) and other interventionists who are similarly guided by attachment theory and research (Heinicke, 1991; Lieberman & Pawl, 1993; Osofsky, Culp, & Ware, 1988).

The birth of a baby and the first few weeks of interaction between parent and child are often a trigger for old feelings. Thus we use this window of opportunity to begin to encourage the parents to link the baby's experience to their own early memories. For example, we might say, "Isn't it amazing how relieved and relaxed your baby seems when you pick him up? Does holding your baby ever make you remember (or wonder) about what it was like for you when you were little and needed someone to hold you?" Or we might draw upon our own experience and comment, "Sometimes when I need to care for my child, I find myself wishing that someone would care for me that way too. Do you have those feelings sometimes?"

For many parents, the demands of caring for a new baby may activate their own feelings of sadness and loss because they have never really felt cared for. In our experience, some parents will (if given permission and acceptance from the facilitator and/or other group members) acknowledge some resentment that they are expected to respond to their babies in a way that no one ever did for them, which represents a kind of jealousy or rivalry with the baby. Bringing such emotions into conscious awareness can be the first step toward letting go of those feelings so that they do not interfere with the parent's ability to respond to the baby.

For some parents, the group is a good place to examine memories from their own childhood, facilitated by the discovery that others have had similar experiences and feelings. In one activity, we put out on a table an array of messages that we might have heard from our parents (in words or actions) when we were growing up. Each mother chooses the messages that she remembers hearing or writes her own on blank cards. The facilitator then encourages mothers to remember and talk about how it felt to experience those messages: good, bad, and everything in between. This can be a painful process, but a useful one for tapping into emotional memories. Next, the mothers are asked to choose messages they wish they had heard in their childhood. Then they are asked to think about which messages they want to pass on to their own child, tearing up the painful ones and keeping the positive ones. At that point in the exercise, mothers and babies move into a free-play time, with the mothers charged with practicing how to give those positive messages to their babies through words and behavior.

PROFESSIONAL BOUNDARIES
AND SELF-REVELATION IN INTERVENTION

The issues we have been discussing in these last sections take us into challenging psychological areas of a parent's life, thoughts, and feelings. This is common ground for psychotherapists or other professionals with extensive training in mental health issues, but for many early intervention practitioners, this can be uncomfortable territory. It is important to remember that parent education is as emotional an experience as it is intellectual, and we must not be afraid of emotion per se. It is imperative, however, that we all work within our areas of competence, and that we seek consultation to assist us with difficult situations and/or that we refer a family out for other therapeutic services as needed.

Nonetheless, there is therapeutic value in sharing the journey with parents by listening empathically, asking questions that encourage them to be self-reflective, and, at times, sharing our own personal stories in a way that supports and encourages the families we serve. (In some mental health professions, this personal sharing is discouraged, but we have found that the advantages outweigh the disadvantages when it is done carefully, sensitively, and on a limited basis.)

Based on our own collective experiences in early intervention across the various settings in which we have worked, we have these observations about effective ways to maintain healthy boundaries even as we enter into a relatively open, personal relationship with the families we serve:

• Parents have found it reassuring and helpful when we occasionally share brief anecdotes about our own challenging parenting experiences and/or the things we wish we'd done differently. This needs to be done in the spirit of emphasizing that none of us is perfect and that, throughout our adult life, we can learn from our mistakes.

• It is fine to share examples of tactics that have worked for us in our own parenting, but such an example should be offered as one of many options from which a family might choose as they seek a solution tailored to their own strengths and needs. (The families might offer some suggestions that help us in our own parenting!)

• When we share personal stories, we need to avoid details that would be embarrassing to our own family members or that betray a confidence we should keep within our own personal network. We also need to avoid intimate details that could make our program participants uncomfortable (e.g., details about a conflict with a spouse).

• In telling personal stories, our goal should always be to advance the learning of the parents we serve, not to get sympathy or affirmation for ourselves. The focus is on our clients' needs, not our own.

• When we use a style of service that includes personal revelation, sometimes program participants will begin to think of us as just friends, losing sight of the professional service relationship. This may lead to invitations to get together on weekends or to attend special events in the life of the family. It is important to think proactively about how to respond to such invitations. For example, program policy might be that it is acceptable for workers to attend a participant's wedding or baby shower if they wish. During the course of a home visit, it might be appropriate occasionally to go out for coffee or lunch, being careful to tie the conversation to the family's program goals. However, a social get-together for a movie or dinner would violate appropriate professional boundaries. Whatever policies are set, it is important to be prepared to explain them clearly to program participants and to clarify boundaries as necessary over the course of working with a family.

SUMMARY

Knowledge, attitudes, beliefs, and expectations underlie all parenting behavior. From the most basic knowledge of developmental milestones, to the deepest understanding of why infants and toddlers behave as they do, these cognitive factors are a major key to optimal parenting and healthy child development. Thus promoting parental knowledge and encouraging an ongoing quest for understanding are central to the early intervention enterprise. At the heart of this work is the goal of enabling parents to see through the eyes of the child, in the hopes that good perspective taking will lead to behavior that is well attuned to the child's feelings and needs.

Yet, even among the most knowledgeable parents, there are often barriers to using that information and translating it into day-to-day parenting practices. One barrier, which has been the focus of extensive research and intervention, is the emotional baggage that comes from parents' lack of resolution about painful experiences in their own childhood. As described in this chapter, research on intergenerational cycles of parenting helps to set some direction for intervention aimed at encouraging parents to examine their past and choose what to carry forward and what to leave behind.

As parents begin to confront the internal factors that support or hinder them in their relationships with their children, they need to muster all available resources to help them in that process. With that in mind, we now turn in Chapter 5 to a discussion of external factors that influence the parent–child relationship and, in particular, the importance of social support in the lives of families with young children.

REFERENCES

Ainsworth, M. D. S., Blehar, M. C., Waters, E., & Wall, S. (1978). *Patterns of attachment: A psychological study of the Strange Situation*. Hillsdale, NJ: Erlbaum.

Brazelton, T. B. (1973). *Neonatal Behavioral Assessment Scale*. Philadelphia: Lippincott.

Breger, L. (1974). *From instinct to identity: The development of personality*. Englewood Cliffs, NJ: Prentice-Hall.

Cardone, I. A., & Gilkerson, L. (1992). Family Administered Neonatal Activities: An adaptation for parents of infants born with Down syndrome. *Infants and Young Children, 5*, 40–48.

Carter, S., Osofsky, J., & Hann, D. M. (1991). Speaking for baby: Therapeutic interventions with adolescent mothers and their infants. *Infant Mental Health Journal, 12*, 291–301.

Christenson, S., & Conoley, J. C. (Eds.). (1992). *Home–school collaboration: Enhancing children's academic and social competence*. Silver Spring, MD: National Association of School Psychologists.

Egeland, B. (1988). Breaking the cycle of abuse: Implications for prediction and intervention. In K. D. Browne, C. Davies, & P. Stratton (Eds.), *Early prediction and prevention of child abuse* (pp. 87–99). New York: Wiley.

Egeland, B., & Breitenbucher, M. (1980). *Final report: The effects of parental knowledge and expectations on the development of child competence* (Grant No. 90-C-1259). Washington, DC: Administration for Children, Youth and Families, Office of Child Development, Department of Health, Education and Welfare.

Erickson, M. F., Korfmacher, J., & Egeland, B. (1992). Attachments past and present: Implications for therapeutic intervention with mother–infant dyads. *Development and Psychopathology, 4*, 495–507.

Erickson, M. F., & Simon, J. (1999). *Steps toward effective, enjoyable parenting: Facilitators' guide*. Minneapolis: Irving B. Harris Training Center for Infant and Toddler Development, University of Minnesota.

Erickson, M. F., Sroufe, L. A., & Egeland, B. (1985). The relationship between quality of attachment and behavior problems in preschool in a high-risk sample. In I. Bretherton & E. Waters (Eds.), Growing points of attachment theory and research. *Monographs of the Society for Research in Child Development, 50*(1–2, Serial No. 209), 147–166.

Fonagy, P., Steele, H., & Steele, M. (1991). Maternal representations of attachment during pregnancy predict the organization of infant–mother attachment at 1 year of age. *Child Development, 62,* 891–905.

Fraiberg, L. (Ed.). (1987). *Selected writings of Selma Fraiberg.* Columbus: Ohio State University Press.

Gunnar, M., Malone, S., & Fisch, R. (1985). The psychobiology of stress and coping in the human neonate: Studies of adrenocortical activity in response to stress in the first week of life. In T. Field, P. McCabe, & N. Schneiderman (Eds.), *Stress and coping* (Vol. 1, pp. 179–196). Hillsdale, NJ: Erlbaum.

Heinicke, C. M. (1991). Early family intervention: Focusing on the mother's adaptation-competence and quality of partnership. In D. G. Unger & D. R. Power (Eds.), *Families as nurturing systems: Support across the life span* (pp. 127–142). New York: Haworth.

Lieberman, A. F., & Pawl, J. H. (1993). Infant–parent psychotherapy. In C. H. Zeanah, Jr. (Ed.), *Handbook of infant mental health* (pp. 427–442). New York: Guilford Press.

Meltzoff, A. N., & Moore, M. K. (1983). Newborn infants imitate adult facial gestures. *Child Development, 54,* 702–709.

Moses, K. (1988). *Lost dreams and growth, parents' concerns: Video presentation and interaction with parents of impaired children* [Video]. Evanston, IL: Resources Networks.

Newberger, C. M. (1980). *Parental Awareness Scoring Manual.* Boston: Children's Hospital.

Newberger, C. M., & Cook, S. J. (1983). Parental awareness and child abuse: A cognitive–developmental analysis of urban and rural samples. *American Journal of Orthopsychiatry, 53,* 512–524.

Nugent, K. J. (1985). *Using the NBAS with infants and their families: Guidelines for intervention.* New York: March of Dimes.

Osofsky, J., Culp, A. M., & Ware, L. M. (1988). Intervention challenges with adolescent mothers and their infants. *Psychiatry, 51,* 236–241.

Piaget, J. (1952). *The origins of intelligence in children.* New York: International Universities Press.

Posada, G., Waters, E., Crowell, J. A., & Lay, K. L. (1995). Is it easier to use a secure mother as a secure base?: Attachment Q-sort correlates of the adult attachment interview. In E. Waters, B. E. Vaughn, G. Posada, & K. Kondo-Ikemura (Eds.), Caregiving, cultural, and cognitive perspectives on secure-base behavior and working models: New growing points of attachment theory and research. *Monographs of the Society for Research in Child Development, 60*(2–3, Serial No. 244), 133–145.

Ricks, M. H. (1985). The social transmission of parental behaviors: Attachment across generations. In E. Bretherton & E. Waters (Eds.), Growing points of attachment theory and research. *Monographs of the Society for Research in Child Development, 50*(1–2, Serial No. 209), 211–227.

Sameroff, A. J., & Feil, L. A. (1985). Parental concepts of development. In I. E. Sigel (Ed.), *Parental belief systems: The psychological consequences for children* (pp. 83–105). Hillsdale, NJ: Erlbaum.

Sroufe, L. A., Fox, N., & Pancake, V. (1983). Attachment and dependency in developmental perspective. *Child Development, 54,* 1615–1627.

FIVE

Strengthening Family Support Networks

Hannah had become pregnant as a teenager and had two young children. She was married to an abusive man, and her older sister Susan became increasingly concerned when Hannah reported that her husband had begun hitting their children as well as her. Over time, Susan convinced her sister to leave the marriage and move over 800 miles to live with her. When Hannah arrived with her children, she was depressed and withdrawn. Her toddler-age son was also withdrawn, and her 6-year-old daughter was angry and acting out. With a lot of effort, Susan managed to enroll her niece in a good public school and connect her sister with the various health and social services for which she was eligible. In turn, Hannah helped out Susan, a single parent, by having a hot meal and neat house waiting for Susan and her preschool-age daughter when they arrived home from work and day care.

Eventually, Susan helped Hannah and her children find subsidized housing into which they moved to ease the crowded conditions in Susan's home. Susan persuaded Hannah to join a parent education program that included her younger child, and eventually Hannah got a job as a child care assistant in the program. Her depression improved, and her children are doing better.

Hannah was fortunate to have a supportive and resourceful sister to turn to when she needed help. Many parents in similar circumstances have no relatives or friends with whom they are closely connected, or, if they are connected to others, these connections may be neither supportive nor helpful. In fact, these connections may be negative influences on an individual or family attempting to grow and change in positive directions. When a person's social connections are with drinking friends who discourage one from sobriety, a negative and interfering mother or in-law who undermines one's self-confidence as a parent, or a controlling partner who is emotionally and/or physically abusive and damages one's sense of self, these connections are not supportive.

There is a wealth of research on the importance of social support to the healthy functioning of families. Bronfenbrenner (1987) reports that the capacity of families to function effectively, particularly under stress, depends to a significant degree on the availability and provision of social support from persons outside the immediate family, such as kin, friends, neighbors, and coworkers. Social support is defined here as resources (e.g., emotional encouragement, potentially useful information, services, or goods) provided to individuals or families in response to the need for assistance (Dunst, Trivette, & Deal, 1988).

A distinction is often made between *informal* and *formal* social support systems. A family's informal social support sources may include relatives, friends, neighbors, coworkers, local business owners, clergy-persons, congregations, libraries, parks, and social clubs. Potential sources of formal social support for families may include organized systems such as child care, schools, social work, health departments, and community-based family support and education programs. Whether formal or informal, however, research shows clearly that social support,

> especially aid and assistance that match family identified needs, enhances parent and family well-being, decreases time demands placed upon a family by a disabled or at-risk child, promotes positive caregiver interactive styles, decreases the display of interfering caregiver interactive styles, enhances positive parental perception of child functioning, and indirectly influences a number of child behavior characteristics, including affect, temperament, and motivation. (Dunst & Trivette, 1990, p. 327)

In Chapters 3 and 4, we focused our intervention strategies primarily on parents and the parent–child relationship. In his ecology of human development framework, Bronfenbrenner (1979) describes a child's growth as occurring within a series of nested systems: the *microsystem, mesosystem, exosystem,* and *macrosystem.* The microsystem includes the face-to-face contacts between children and their immediate environment, such as family, school, church, and peers. The mesosystem is the composite of the microsystems with which an individual regularly interacts. Exosystems are social structures in which children may not directly participate, but that strongly influence the quality of family life and child development, such as workplaces, mass media, and local government. Macrosystems are the larger cultural and institutional influences on child development, such as political and economic systems. This chapter moves out from the parent and parent–child focus of earlier chapters to look at strengthening family support networks throughout these systems, with particular focus on mesosytems and exosystems.

BASIC PRINCIPLES OF FAMILY SUPPORT

National attention to the need for family support has risen significantly since the late 1970s when family resource programs began to proliferate across the country. Often beginning in a neighborhood-based agency or as federal or state pilot efforts, these programs were responding to families' needs for information and support. The services they offered included resource referral, parent education, service access and coordination, child development information or educational child care, and life-skills training. Their roots were in the settlement houses of the late 1800s to early 1900s and in self-help groups. Yet their approach to serving families was qualitatively different from these earlier efforts and stressed prevention, promotion of healthy behaviors, and empowerment. A professional organization, the Family Resource Coalition of America, was formed in the early 1980s in direct response to this growth of family resource programs and currently serves as a networking and advocacy arm for members nationwide (Weissbourd, 1987).

In 1991, the Family Resource Coalition of America published its summary of guiding principles of family support that had evolved over 10 years of work with programs (Pooley, 1994, p. 5). First, "The basic relationship between program and family is one of equality and respect; the program's first priority is to establish and maintain this relationship as the vehicle through which growth and change can occur" (p. 5). Just as relationships determine the quality of connections between parents and children, students and teachers, clergy and congregation, and most of our human social interactions, so they are central to the effectiveness of programs with participating families.

Second, "Participants are a vital resource; programs facilitate parents' ability to serve as resources to each other, to participate in program decisions and governance, and to advocate for themselves in the community" (Pooley, 1994, p. 5). Parents have much to teach to and learn from each other. Participation and advocacy mean that staff encourage parents to act on their own behalf in shaping the content and style of program services, and in enhancing the "family-friendliness" of the communities in which they live and work.

Third, "Programs are community based and culturally and socially relevant to the families they serve; programs are often a bridge between families and other services outside the scope of the program" (Pooley, 1994, p. 5). To increase their accessibility and utility for participants, programs are located within communities of residence, employment, or other affiliation. Programs work actively to increase their cultural competence, as described later in this chapter, in order to be more inclusive and useful for the families in their communities. Staff help families to find and use other formal and informal support resources in addition to those provided by the program.

Fourth, "Parent education, information about human development, and skill building for parents are essential parts of every program" (Pooley, 1994, p. 5). It is amazing that the most important and challenging task for many of us, the raising of our children, is a task for which we are often so unprepared and so "unsupported" as we go along. Although parents can find advice in a wide spectrum of places, from pediatricians, to glossy magazines, to bookstores' loaded shelves, to television talk shows, to newspaper columnists, to churches, this advice is usually contradictory and not always developmentally or culturally appropriate. Family support programs offer parent education and skill building as essential services to all parents.

Fifth, and finally, "Programs are voluntary, and seeking support and information is viewed as a sign of family strength, not as an indication of deficits and problems" (Pooley, 1994, p. 5). Because all parents need information and support, acknowledging this need is a positive statement, not an admission of weakness. Just as most of us do not appreciate advice or help that is forced upon us, most families are interested primarily in services that are voluntary, that they can elect to use or not. The key to gaining their participation is in making programs and/or services useful, culturally appropriate, accessible, and attractive, and in actively recruiting the families we seek to serve.

Underlying these principles are some important assumptions. The Family Resource Coalition (Pooley, 1994, p. 6) asserts that all family support programs are grounded in the following premises:

- Families have primary responsibility for their children's development and well-being; they need resources and supports that will enable them to fulfill that responsibility effectively.
- Healthy families are the foundation of a healthy society. Families who are unable to promote their children's development ultimately place the entire society at risk.
- Families operate as part of a total system. Children cannot be viewed as separate from their families, nor can families be viewed

separately from their communities, their cultural heritage, or the society at large. Decisions made on behalf of children must consider the ways in which these various systems are interconnected.

- The systems and institutions upon which families rely for support must assist families' efforts to effectively raise their children. They must adjust and coordinate their services so as not to hinder families' abilities to maintain positive environments for their children.

These principles and assumptions should remain at the foreground of our consciousness as we plan, implement, evaluate, and revise family services and programs. As these principles are fully integrated into our work, its quality and utility for families will be radically transformed for the better.

POWER: OLD MYTHS AND NEW INSIGHTS

As we think about notions of support and help giving, it is important to consider issues of power, which are implicit in several of the principles discussed above. Throughout this chapter and book, we use words like *community, relationships, support, empowering, reform, resources,* and so forth. At a basic level, all of these terms are related to power: its definition, its uses, and its potential. In *The Quickening of America,* Lappe and DuBois (1994) discuss the concept of power in terms of myths that limit and insights that empower. Three sets of these will be examined here as they relate to working with families and children.

1. The Limiting Myth: Power is evil. It's always corrupting. It's always used by a few power holders to block change that benefits others. To be good people, we should avoid power.

   The Empowering Insight: We cannot realize our values or goals without power. Power is the capacity to act publicly and effectively, to bring about positive change, to build hope. (Lappe & DuBois, 1994, p. 47)

When families and interventionists focus on problem solving, it becomes obvious that power is not something to condemn or avoid. In order to solve complex problems, families need to work in partnership with interventionists, rather than being passive recipients of services. Cynicism is grounded in feelings of powerlessness. Families need opportunities to exercise real power over their circumstances. Power will then shift to a more equitable equilibrium between interventionists and families, with both workers and families as the winners. Family workers will find their efforts to be more productive and satisfying, and families will enhance their sense of competence and control. The positive change that is likely to result will build hope on all sides.

> 2. The Limiting Myth: Since there's only so much of it around, the more power you have, the less there is for me.
>
> The Empowering Insight: Relational power expands possibilities for many people at once. The more you use it, the more there is. (Lappe & DuBois, 1994, p. 48)

Lappe and DuBois discuss a concept called *relational power*. This view holds that power is not a fixed advantage to be contested. It is about human capacity to do things. These capacities can only be developed with others. Thus power can expand for many people simultaneously (1994, pp. 48–49). This is a radical change from our society's common view that "the bigger the pie piece you get, the smaller the piece I get." It is a paradox that power that is withheld will shrink, while power that is shared will expand. What this means for interventionists is that they will not lose or diminish their power by sharing it with the families they serve. Instead, in terms of their effectiveness and ability to get things done, their power will expand in direct proportion to the degree their client families are empowered.

> 3. The Limiting Myth: Power is a one-way force over someone. It means that you're in control and can get others to do what you want.
>
> The Empowering Insight: Power always exists in relationships, going both ways. In relationships, the actions of each affect the other, so no one is ever completely powerless. (Lappe & DuBois, 1994, p. 51)

Many interventionists are trained in family systems theory, which holds that the actions of any one family member affect the actions of the others. If this is true, it follows that no family member is ever completely powerless. In the interventionist–family relationship, this concept also holds. Despite the fact that there are very real power imbalances in our society based on income, gender, race, and other categories, this understanding can be used as a tool by less powerful groups or individuals to work toward more equitable relationships with the more powerful. As interventionists, we can use this understanding to underscore the importance of empowering families and working toward power *with*, rather than *over* them. Adapting Morgaine's (1988) definition of empowerment to our work, it means that family members will increase their belief in their ability to learn and make changes in their family life, their ability to think and act critically with regard to life situations, and their power over negative circumstances (p. 41).

SERVICE COLLABORATION
FOR BETTER FAMILY SUPPORT

As we discussed in Chapter 1, there is currently an increasing emphasis on collaboration among and integration of various interventions and services. Our traditional system of family supports and services is inadequate and largely ineffective as a formal support network for families and children. It does not have the connections among the pieces that define a mesosystem. It does not even merit being called a system. The *American Heritage Dictionary* (1992, p. 1823) defines system as "a group of interacting, interrelated, or interdependent elements forming a complex whole." If our current collection of public and private health, education, and social services, as well as overall public policy, were truly interactive, interrelated, and interdependent, we would have a real system of family support. This three-part definition can serve as an interesting framework for the current emphasis on service collaboration.

Interaction, often referred to as *networking* or *sharing information*, can serve as the initial stage of collaboration. Although providers in health, education, and social services often share the common goal of strengthening families and use similar means to do so, they are typically quite uninformed about each other's activities. The result for many low-income families is that in some areas, they are overserved (resulting in exasperating duplication), whereas other needs are not addressed at all. For example, a low-income single mother of an infant with fetal alcohol syndrome may have three case managers, time-intensive "services" that a less needy parent would reject outright. Yet she may still lack someone to care for her infant when she needs a break from the stress of daily living. If service providers interacted on a regular basis and worked to coordinate their efforts more effectively, this type of misdirected effort would decrease.

Interrelating implies a reciprocal relationship between and among service providers, a next step after interaction. When a family expresses a need to us as interventionists, it is important to do our best to help the family get that need met. However, most professionals are limited as to what they can offer by fiscal and other constraints. In addition to focusing on informal resources within the community, providers can better serve families by bartering with one another. For example, a parent education program can offer an ongoing parent group for families, with transport provided by a van and driver from the local Head Start program. The Head Start program is able to secure high-quality parent education for its clients for a minimal investment of time and money. The parent education program is able to draw families into its center that it might not otherwise reach. Both agencies are winners, with the participating parents and children as beneficiaries.

Interdependence among service providers is the hallmark of true collaboration and probably the most difficult to achieve. Our dominant society considers independence to be one of our most primary values. We value it so much that we often subscribe to child-rearing practices that are contrary to both our infants' needs and to our own instincts, because we feel that these practices will further our own and our children's independence. The irony, however, is that children learn independence from having their early needs met, that is, by being allowed to be dependent in their first years of life. Parents will recover their independence as their children grow up and leave home, sometimes all too soon.

Interdependence implies that two or more parties are dependent on one another. Systems theorists tell us that this mutual dependence is a fact of all life forms. Yet most institutions and many individuals behave as if their actions are independent of those of others. They may even believe that this is a virtue to be sought rather than a problem to be addressed. Effective family interventionists understand that they are mutually dependent on the actions of other service providers, larger societal factors, and the families they serve. This knowledge enables them actively to seek ways of working together with families and other service providers—to do *with,* rather than to do *to* or *for.*

In this society, most institutions, whether they are large, governmental departments of health or small, nonprofit service agencies, tend to be pyramidal in structure with a specified chain of command. This means that if line workers are actively working toward better collaboration with line workers in other agencies without the support or involvement of upper management, their efforts are likely to fail. System reform ventures are apt to work best if they come from both the top down and the bottom up. Yet top-level managers may not be motivated to streamline family services and may, in fact, be prompted to oppose reforms for fear of losing power. Add to this the human tendency to resist change, and it is clear why system reform often collides with inertia. It's possible that line workers, who may gain the most by more efficient service delivery, will need to build their critical mass along with their clients until the reform voices are too loud to ignore. See Kagan (1991) and Winer and Ray (1994) in the resource bibliography at the end of the book for information on improving collaboration in order to provide better service to families and children.

A RESOURCE-BASED APPROACH
TO WORKING WITH FAMILIES

To counter the increasing social problems emerging in our modern society, and recognizing the decrease in funds for social services, current literature alludes to the importance of a resource-based rather than a service-based approach to providing social support to families (Dunst, Trivette, & Deal, 1994). *Service* is defined as "a specific or particular activity employed by a professional or professional agency for rendering help or assistance to an individual or group." *Resources* are defined as "the full range of possible types of community help or assistance that might be mobilized and used to meet the needs of an individual or group" (p. 141).

Fundamental to respectful help for families is the assumption that the family and not a helping professional must define the need for assistance (Pilusuk & Parks, 1986). The family also chooses where, how, and when to use this help. Reflecting on our own experience, we are more likely to be receptive to support when we have sought it, rather than when it is pushed upon us. The appropriate role of formal service systems is seen as identifying, supplementing, and expanding a family's resources for informal social support. Hobbs et al. (1984) assert that when we professionalize all types of family services, we interfere with and often preclude a family's opportunities to identify and strengthen more naturally occurring support networks.

All families require resources and support for healthy and stable functioning. The terms *resource rich* and *resource poor* reflect the notion that families differ more in their access to resources (not exclusively monetary) than they do in their basic goals and aspirations. Helping families identify and expand these resources is an appropriate and effective focus for human service workers. It's also more productive than always providing direct service, because resource-based approaches to working with families have a wider range of possibilities than fiscally constrained service-based approaches (Katz, 1984). Expanding resources also goes beyond treating or preventing pathology toward promoting healthy functioning. When family members identify their needs, assets, and sources of support, they're exhibiting recognized traits of healthy families (Curran, 1983).

Assessing Family Support Resources

To identify current and needed resources with families, a framework is useful. Dunst et al. (1994) identify 12 categories of resources required by all families:

- Economic (money for necessities and emergencies).
- Physical and environmental (adequate housing, safe neighborhood).
- Food and clothing (food for at least two meals a day, enough clothes for each season).

- Medical and dental care (availability of general and emergency medical and dental care).
- Vocational (opportunity to work, satisfaction with work).
- Transportation and communication (means of getting where one needs to go and for contacting relatives and friends).
- Adult education (available and accessible educational opportunities as needed).
- Child education (opportunities to play with other children, appropriate toys).
- Child care (help in routine daily care, child care while employed).
- Recreational (opportunities for relaxing and fun activities).
- Emotional (sense of belonging to family or group, companionship).
- Cultural and social (opportunities to share value-related experiences with others). (p. 146)

McKnight (1989) suggests four broad social groups that can serve as sources of support for meeting these varied needs. They are (1) personal–social network members, such as spouse or partner, relatives, friends, neighbors, child care providers, or clergypersons; (2) associational groups, such as church groups, interest clubs, self-help groups, block clubs, school groups, or sports leagues; (3) community programs and professionals, such as public or private schools, senior citizen programs, child care centers, libraries, community colleges, or housing programs; and (4) specialized professional services, such as public health clinics, early intervention programs, family preservation programs, substance abuse programs, or respite care.

Identifying a family's supportive resources can be accomplished through *interviews, self-reports,* or *observations.* When interviewing families, helpgivers can use the communication techniques described later in this chapter. Beginning with the underlying assumption that every family has assets and resources, the interviewer will focus on helping families label and describe these. Open-ended questions can be structured around categories such as those described above (Dunst et al., 1994; McKnight, 1989).

For example, we can ask a family, "What kind of child care arrangements are you able to make for your child when you go to work? What about when your child is sick? What kind of information have you gotten from using the child care resource and referral phone number? Which friends or relatives nearby might be able to help with child care?"

To use self-report, we can create instruments that will ask for information to help families identify their needs and resources. Useful scales have been created by Dunst, Trivette, and Deal (1988) and are available in that book's appendices or as a separate packet (ask for full-size scales for *Enabling and Empowering Families*) from the publisher. Whatever forms we ask parents to fill out, we must make special efforts to (1) ask only for information that we will use, (2) use forms that are clear and easy to read and answer, and (3) keep the completed forms confidential.

When we use observation to help families identify their resources and sources of support, some basic principles apply. If we observe families in our programs, we must be sensitive to their possible discomfort and lack of familiarity with the environment. If we observe families in their homes or communities, it is wise to assume the role of a mannerly guest and show respect and appreciation for their hospitality. In all cases, we must be conscious of observing as objectively as possible. Awareness of one's own biases and values, a topic that will be discussed later in this chapter, will go a long way toward better objectivity during observation. Taking notes while watching children at play is a good way to work on observation skills. We can examine our notes and learn to distinguish between *what* we have seen (objectivity) and our *interpretation* of what we have seen (subjectivity).

Regardless of how we collect information to help families identify their needs and resources, an essential final step is verifying accuracy with the families themselves. Noticing body language during interviews, self-report completion, or observations and asking clarifying questions will help to accomplish this. We want to be sure that families are satisfied that the information collected reflects their situation appropriately.

Effective Resource-Based Helping Skills

Working with families to assess their strengths and needed resources is an essential early step in effective interventions. But what about the quality of these parent–helpgiver interactions? If we are working as partners with parents, this requires different helping skills than we may use in the role of professionals as "experts." Although some of these skills are taught in preservice training programs for interventionists, some are not. Let's consider them as they apply to a resource-based perspective, versus one that is service based.

As in most human encounters, building a trusting relationship is basic to effective professional interaction with families. Klass (1996) asserts that development occurs within and through relationships, and that all relationships involve mutuality. Remembering that everyone has something to teach and everyone has something to learn will help to avoid the "helpgiver as expert, parent as passive client" syndrome. We are usually quite put out if friends or strangers make judgmental remarks about our parenting abilities. Why should the parents we work with be any different? Looking for each family's existing and potential resources requires an open mind and respectful attitude, which are basic elements of a trusting relationship.

Effective communication may be the most important characteristic of all. It depends in large part on *careful and attentive listening*, with the listener responding empathically to the speaker and reflecting back what he or she hears to make certain it is what the speaker meant to say. It means really tuning in to what another person is saying, not just mentally rehearsing the next remark while watching the other person's lips move. It consists of asking open questions, which tend to elicit longer responses, instead of closed ones, which tend to invoke yes, no, and other one-word answers. For example, "What are your baby's usual night sleep patterns?" is an open question; "Does your baby sleep through the night?" is a closed one. *Choosing our words carefully in delicate situations* so that they are as objective and noninflammatory as possible is another essential tool of good communication. For example, instead of saying, "I think yanking your child's arm like that is abusive," we could try, "It's really hard when your baby has a tantrum in a public place. Is there any way I can help?"

Being respectful of families means seeking only that information relevant to concerns being addressed and no more. Using "one-size-fits-all" forms that request exhaustive amounts of information on all families is not appropriate. Any standard intake forms should be as simple and brief as possible, with other information sought only as needed. Sometimes the questions asked on standard forms currently used by human service providers are intrusive and may be irrelevant to the support or service requested by the family. Health, education, and social service providers must work together to streamline intake forms and procedures. In constructing questions and forms, it can be helpful to ask ourselves if we would feel comfortable responding to these items.

Often interventionists have been trained to look for the causes of problems rather than focusing on solutions. It certainly is pertinent to ask families what they identify as the reasons for their concerns. Yet probing beyond that to verify if we agree with their assessment is often intrusive and nonproductive. Frequently the solutions are similar regardless of the cause. When we focus on jointly identifying solutions with families to resolve or improve a situation, we are modeling an active approach to problem solving that is not shaming or demeaning of families. Working toward solutions also expands a family's sense of internal locus of control and competence.

This action focus must be balanced, however, with allowing parents time to vent their frustrations. In one school, a teacher will occasionally approach another and say, "Can I whine to you for a while about . . . ?" The second teacher listens sympathetically, and the first may come up with his or her own solution or often just says, "Thanks for listening. I feel better now." Sometimes parents just need to know that someone has heard them.

Finally, as has always been true, giving effective help requires clear assurance of ongoing confidentiality. On those occasions when service providers feel compelled to share information about a family with other professionals, they must first seek written permission from the family, specifying clearly *what* information is to be shared, *why,* and with *whom.* Once approval is granted, helpgivers are bound to honor this agreement. It may be necessary to revisit the specifics of the agreement periodically to ensure that they are current.

In a group situation, such as an ongoing parent discussion group, confidentiality means that all members acknowledge that what is said in the group stays in the group. For example, if one parent admits to losing his temper with his child, he should not have to worry that it will be spread around his workplace or neighborhood by other group partici-pants. The only exception to this rule should be when there are grounds to suspect abuse. In these situations, group leaders are ethically and legally bound to report their suspicions to a child protection profes-sional. The facilitator should alert the group to this reporting responsi-bility in one of the first group meetings.

On reflection, most of us desire or demand all of these qualities in our interactions with helpgivers around our own problem or issues, whether the helpgivers are relatives, friends, partners, or service provid-ers. Why should we assume that the families with whom we work deserve any less?

BARRIERS TO USING RESOURCES
AND STRATEGIES TO ADDRESS THESE BARRIERS

Sometimes, although there may be many resources available to families, parents cannot or do not use them. Whether we work with families in their homes or in our centers, we can help them build the skills to seek and accept support from others in their families and communities. The first step is for family members to recognize and acknowledge that they have needs. The saying "Children's needs are best met by adults whose needs are met" (author unknown) can be posted in our written materials and our centers, and modeled by practitioners.

Once a family asserts its normalcy by recognizing its needs, we can discuss getting the resources to meet these needs. One question to pose early in the conversation is "What keeps you from getting support/help for ... ?" Although the responses will be as varied as the families we ask, let's look at some typical barriers to using supportive resources and strategies to address these barriers.

Lack of Information about Resources

To promote family skills and confidence for using formal community resources, practitioners can begin by providing parents with clear information about available resources and services. A simple community directory that is printed as inexpensively as possible, while still being clear and attractive, will make it easier to revise and reprint the directory as necessary. In some areas, organizations such as the United Way may have an information and referral service that is accessed by dialing a single telephone number. Regardless of their field, all practitioners should consider it their professional obligation to remain informed and current about related resources and services that may be of value to their clients. Information, resources, and referrals must be essential parts of any program serving families.

Lack of Skill or Confidence to Access Resources

Possession of resource information does not always predict access. Interventionists may need to coach parents to ask pertinent questions and possibly have parents role play asking the questions by telephone and in person. Some important questions include the following:

- Who is eligible for this service or program?
- What does it offer?
- What does it cost?
- What is the application process?
- Are there any time limits on this service or program?
- If there is a waiting list, how long does it take to become a participant?
- How could I speak with someone who has used your program or service?
- How can I apply or get on the waiting list?
- Does your program or service have any transportation or child care assistance for participants?

Even when thinking about informal sources of support (e.g., family and friends), parents sometimes are unsure how to ask for assistance. Again, role play can help.

Old Messages That Get in the Way

Some adults have received lots of negative messages as children such as "You always mess things up. You'll never amount to anything. You're just like . . . (someone disliked and not respected). Stop crying, or I'll give you something to cry about. Why can't you be more like your sister? You asked for that." Clues that parents may be haunted by negative childhood messages may be revealed in statements such as "I don't want to bother anyone," "I should be able to do this on my own," or "I can never do anything right."

Remembering some of these long-lasting messages and how they made us feel can help us overcome their effects on our adult lives. As discussed in Chapter 4, group discussion can be an effective way to process them and substitute more positive messages for ourselves and our children. Examples of positive messages include "Everyone makes mistakes." "I'm sure you'll be able to make the right decision for you and your baby." "We all have times when we need to ask for help." "You'll do well." "I'm sorry that happened to you." "Can I help you find a ride to the clinic?" In our groups or one-on-one work, we need to emphasize that *all* adults and children have the right to ask for help and support, make mistakes, change their minds, and say "No."

Lack of Problem-Solving Skills

When difficult life issues overwhelm parents or simple lack of experience inhibits them, we can work with them on developing problem-solving skills. Focusing on a barrier or complaint that parents identify, we can work through the following steps. It often helps to write down responses during the process.

1. Identify the problem. What's the issue? Whose problem is it?
2. Gather information about the problem, both the facts and personal feelings about and reactions to these facts.
3. Generate a list of possible solutions to the problem. Be creative here, and don't hold back.
4. Choose a few favorite solutions. List and evaluate the pros and cons of each.
5. Select one solution to try. If it works, congratulations are in order. If it doesn't work, try another.

Resistance to Advice

Some individuals resist any responses to their requests for help by arguing, "Yes . . . but . . . ," or "I tried that and it didn't work." Parents with an external locus of control may be especially prone to this behavior. It's often helpful in these situations (and in general) to avoid saying anything that may be construed as advice. When parents complain about an issue and ask for ideas on what to do, we can respond, "What have you tried?" When parents answer, we listen sympathetically and respond, "How did that work for you? What else have you tried?"

After the conversation has warmed up, parents will often come up with their own solutions and/or be more receptive to statements such as "It sounds like that worked well for you. . . . Have you ever thought about . . . ? Have you ever tried . . . ?" In any event, using this approach is more respectful of parents' competence and autonomy and thus is generally more acceptable than giving direct advice.

Uncertainty about Goals

Parents who have grown up and/or are now living in chaotic environments may have little experience in setting and achieving goals. This requires a future orientation that is difficult for people who are focused on day-to-day survival. Interventionists can work with parents on setting a few simple goals and breaking down their achievement into small, manageable steps. Despite apparent willingness to work toward a goal, parents may occasionally appear ambivalent. When this occurs, it may be helpful to examine possible unanticipated consequences of achieving a goal and look for ways to deal with them.

For example, a young teen mother may say that she is intent on finishing high school. Yet she appears to be undermining her own efforts in that direction by cutting classes regularly. When probed, she reveals that her mother, with whom she and her baby are now living, has told her that when she graduates, she must find a place of her own to live. Because this is a frightening prospect to her, the young mother is not able to commit fully to her goal of graduating. She may need help in anticipating and handling this issue in order for her to accomplish her goal.

Lack of Conflict Resolution Skills

Most of us are wary of conflict and may be unaware of how we tend to deal with it. We may also not know that there are a variety of ways of dealing with conflict. None of these ways is necessarily right or wrong. They include the following:

- Fighting to the death.
- Walking away.
- Giving in totally.

- Compromising: "I'll do x if you do y."
- Helping everyone "win."

For example, if a stranger grabs our toddler from our side in a shopping mall, we would scream and struggle mightily until our child was safe. If we come upon two people in a fist fight on a street corner, we may quickly cross the street and call 911 from a safe distance. If we are about to force our child to change her selection of green plaid pants and purple striped shirt, we may recognize that it's not really important and allow her to wear her mismatched outfit. If we argue with our partner about housework, we may suggest that we do the dishes if he or she does the cooking. When something in our family is not working well, we may try a family discussion in which everyone gets a chance both to complain and to contribute solutions.

These situations illustrate five very different ways of handling conflict. Yet for each situation, the response may be the best one. The point is that there is no one right way to deal with conflict. If we are stuck using only one or two of these responses in every situation, we may want to broaden our repertoire. Role playing or practicing different ways of reacting to different predicaments can be very helpful if done with a delicate sense of humor in a safe environment where people know and trust each other.

Lack of Communication Skills

Learning techniques of assertive communication will enhance the ability of parents to acquire needed support. Interventionists can work with both adults and children on skills such as the following:

- Recognizing and expressing feelings accurately and verbally.
- Using "I" messages ("When you do x, I feel y").
- Saying "No" to inappropriate demands (reinforcement here may be needed especially by women).
- Avoiding name calling and absolute statements ("You're such a. . . . " "You never. . . . ").
- Substituting direct messages for *triangulation* (triangulation being when A has a problem with B and speaks to C about it instead of directly to B).
- Asking for what is needed.

In order to use these skills successfully, individuals must feel confident and worthwhile enough to risk these modes of direct communication. If they have very negative working models of themselves, they may first need to address these with skilled mental health professionals. Other interventionists can simultaneously help parents to contradict these negative working models through awareness, modeling, persistence, and patience.

HOME VISITING AS A FAMILY
SUPPORT STRATEGY

In addition to the barriers described above, there are more basic barriers to families using center-based resources and services. Because of transportation or child care issues, or due to stress and physical and/or social isolation, some families may not be able or willing to come into a group or center location, at least not initially. In these instances, family-friendly agencies will provide home visits.

For example, the Prenatal/Early Infancy Project accomplished important benefits for children and mothers in a semirural area of New York State, when nurses made home visits prenatally and in the first 2 years of a child's life (Olds, Henderson, Tatelbaum, & Chamberlin, 1988). Or, as in the case of the STEEP program described in earlier chapters, home visits can be a way to engage participants personally in a group program and/or to adapt group activities to unique individuals and families.

Weiss, of the Harvard Family Research Project, describes home visits as a "necessary but not sufficient" component of all programs for families and children (Weiss, 1993, p. 113). They are necessary because of the features that distinguish them from center-based services. First, by definition, home visits take place in a family's home. This enables a practitioner to reach isolated families who would not come to a center, to gain an ecological perspective of the family's situation, and to help equalize the power imbalance between parent and practitioner. Second, the one-on-one contact of home visits is more conducive than center-based approaches to building trusting relationships between parents and program staff. These relationships are a prerequisite for constructive staff–client interactions. Finally, Weiss describes the "linchpin role" of home visitors in assessing families' needs and connecting them to needed services as contributing significantly to program effectiveness (1993, p. 121). This role relates to the responsibility of practitioners, as discussed earlier in this chapter, to remain informed and current about related resources and services.

Home visits are not sufficient, however, because we know that no single program or service approach is enough to support families in and of itself. Nor is our current patchwork of categorical programs and services efficient, cost effective, or accessible for most families. Children and families of all income levels need a comprehensive continuum of family support policies and services. For now, however, well-trained and supervised home visitors can serve as a universal access point for families into existing services.

To be most effective, home visits are set up so that families can tailor their time with us to suit their needs. The STEEP program (Erickson & Simon, 1999) asks mothers to decide issues such as the following:

- *Where* should visitor and parent meet? At her home? A nearby park? At the program office?
- *Who* should be included in the visit besides Mom and baby? Baby's father? Other family members? Friends?
- *How* shall we use this time? Sit and talk? Go out for a walk? Do some laundry? Bathe the baby?

Asking parents to decide the answers to these questions models our belief in their competence and ability to identify their own family's resources and needs.

Home visitors will want to bring a selection of developmentally appropriate toys and activities for the children who will be present in the home. Playing with the children is a good way to break the ice and model effective parent–child interaction strategies. It also gives parents the spoken or unspoken message, "Your child is an interesting person and fun to be with." As discussed at some length in Chapter 3, videotaping is also an excellent activity for focusing on parent and child during home visits. See Wasik, Bryant, and Lyons (1990) and Klass (1996) in the resource bibliography at the end of the book for extensive information on the "what" and "how" of home visiting.

PARENT SUPPORT GROUPS

Although home visits are a powerful intervention strategy, they are less useful for linking parents with other parents and strengthening informal support systems. Parent support groups can fulfill these functions very effectively. Their potential benefits include less social isolation, more appropriate expectations for children, and more competent parenting practices. Powell (1995) suggests that long-term discussion groups are much more effective than direct instruction in changing parental beliefs and practices.

A more subtle, but no less important, potential benefit is the opportunity for parents to help one another. Because the roles of helpgiver and receiver are interchangeable within parent support groups, the helping is rewarding to the giver and nonbinding to the receiver. This reciprocity more closely resembles the healthy give and take of informal support systems such as family and neighbors.

According to a recent national review of parenting programs, there are more than 100,000 parent groups that meet during the course of a year (Carter, 1995). Although these vary widely in sponsorship, orientation, and content, they have in common the reciprocity of parents supporting one another. Carter identifies several essential components of parent groups: *membership, duration and frequency of meetings, content and format, facilitation,* and *sponsorship.*

Membership of parent groups depends in large part on the goals of the group. If the goal is to strengthen families in general, all types of parents are welcome. If the goal is more specific, such as to help teen mothers relate sensitively to their infants and toddlers, those parents would be the targeted group members. In general, when participation in the group is voluntary, as opposed to mandated, members tend to be more committed and involved. However, mandated members may also become invested in the group over time. Parent group size can range from about 6 to 20 members or more. In our experience, the optimal size to offer a variety of perspectives and allow active participation of all members appears to be about 10–12.

Most parent support groups meet from 1 to 3 hours weekly or biweekly over time. If the group members are to establish an essential trust level with one another and the group leader, a minimum suggested number of successive meetings is 4–6. Less than this might be more accurately called a workshop than a parent support group. Evaluation results imply that opportunities for long-term participation should be provided for parents, as changing established parenting behaviors takes time (Cooke, 1992).

Regarding content and format, although there are parent education curricula available, they are best used as helpful resources rather than precise recipes for the parent group meetings. A true support group responds to the needs of its members. Following a previously prescribed sequence of topics and methods without current member input is not likely to accomplish this. It also implies that the group leader has power over the group members, and this power imbalance is not conducive to an effective support group.

Of all the group ingredients, the quality of the facilitation provided by the group leader is probably the most critical. Facilitation is radically different from a lecture–listen approach to teaching and learning. The facilitator must be knowledgeable in group process and able to foster the productive interaction among group members that is integral to support groups. A facilitator who weaves participatory learning strategies into the meeting format will enhance the process further. For example, instead of lecturing on infant nutrition, the facilitator can bring in samples of different types of bottled and frozen baby food, as well as some fresh foods and a baby food grinder. After parents use the baby food grinder, they can do a taste test on all the baby food samples while discussing their nutritional value. In Chapter 4, we discuss several other approaches to participatory group strategies.

Sponsorship of and funding for parent groups includes such diverse sources as federal, state, and county governments; schools; churches; hospitals; drug treatment centers; businesses; private nonprofit agencies; and child care programs. Any of these can work well; it depends on the competence of the facilitators and the training, supervision, and backing they receive from the sponsor. One caution is to be aware of the potential inhibitors or issues a particular sponsor may present. For example, some parents may be reluctant to admit to problems with their children if the parent group is sponsored by their employer and meets at their workplace.

Parent support groups will be more effective if activities for young children of group participants are offered concurrently, with opportunities for parent–child interaction, such as a family meal or shared tasks, offered in the group setting. If parents need to find their own child care in order to attend a parent support group, we are sending a very mixed message indeed. Moreover, it is informative and helpful for all parents, and especially for parents of children with special needs, to see their children interacting with other children of similar age. For example, parents of prematurely born infants will appreciate seeing the similarities of their children with other "premies," as well as discussing common concerns and questions. Parents of hearing-impaired children can learn from watching them interact with other children, both those with disabilities and those without.

The choice of topics for group discussion should be entrusted to the participants. A useful method is to ask parents at the first group meeting what topics they want to discuss. Write the ideas down onto large poster paper as parents state them. If an important topic is not brought up, the facilitator can ask, "Are you interested in talking about . . . ?" Depending on the reaction of the group, this topic can be added to the list and may spur further ideas. The facilitator can type the ideas from the poster paper into a topic list and use it to plan the sessions over the coming weeks. At the end of each group meeting, using topics from this list, the facilitator can suggest, "Next week, we can talk about . . . or. . . . Which would you prefer?" If the group wants to address a new topic not on the list, the facilitator should be responsive to the group's wishes.

A final, but very basic, consideration when planning parent support groups is the atmosphere of the meeting room. Arranging chairs in a circle or using a round table is optimal to enable all parents to see each other's faces clearly and to convey the equal status of all participants. If a circle is not feasible, a square or wide rectangular table is definitely preferable to a long rectangular table where it is almost impossible to see the faces of people seated on the same side. The composition of the group should be considered when selecting room lights. For families of newborns and very young babies, softer, indirect lighting is much more comfortable for the babies than bright overhead lights. Coffee, tea, and water should be always be available, and food can help to create a welcoming atmosphere. Families meeting in the early evening will appreciate being offered a light meal prior to the start of group time. Extensive information and curriculum ideas for parent support groups are provided in the resource bibliography at the end of this book.

BUILDING CULTURAL COMPETENCE

In Ourselves

Whether we approach families through home visits or center-based programs, we know that a family's network of resources and support is determined in part by its cultural context. If we wish to help families identify and expand their support systems, we need to understand something about these contexts. The United States is one of the most ethnically diverse countries in the world. It is composed of many different cultures, each with its own values, beliefs, customs, and behaviors. Yet historically, our major helping systems—health, education, and social services—were built on a European American cultural perspective. The majority of human service professionals were acculturated and trained in this dominant perspective.

Today we realize that using a single cultural lens to focus on a multitude of cultures is clearly inadequate and that, in fact, it can harm rather than help children and families. Lynch and Hanson state, "A cardinal rule in working with all families is to make no assumptions about their concerns, priorities, and resources" (1992, p. 41). We also know that to idealize or vilify any single culture or group of cultures is not helpful. As Garbarino (1995b) notes, "Each culture has something to teach, and each culture has something to learn."

Cross, Bazron, Dennis, and Isaacs (1989) have identified five essential elements for individuals, agencies, or systems to become more culturally competent. The first three of these elements are focused more on our own attitudes, behaviors, and beliefs, while the last two directly address how we do business as interventionists. The first element is to recognize the importance and value of cultural diversity. The *American Heritage Dictionary* (1992) defines culture as "socially transmitted behavior patterns, arts, beliefs, institutions, and all other products of human work and thought" and "these patterns, traits, and products considered as the expression of a particular period, class, community, or population" (p. 454).

It is obvious to thinking persons who have traveled to other parts of the world or spent time with people from other ethnic backgrounds that human cultures differ. Culturally competent persons realize that human cultures are neither better nor worse than one another, but different. This difference is interesting, valuable, and part of what brings texture and complexity to human existence. And although we must recognize and respect our differences, we must not lose sight of the fact that as humans, we are often more alike than different (Campinha-Bacote, 1995).

The second essential element to building cultural competence is to acknowledge and assess continually one's own cultural biases and values. Many Americans of Anglo or European extraction are unaware of their cultural roots. Researching our own racial and ethnic background is important and illuminating. Despite our society's glorification of individualism, we are largely creatures of culture with individual differences. Becoming more aware of how our attitudes, behaviors, and habits are affected by our cultural background is the precursor to becoming more aware of how other people's attitudes, behaviors, and habits may be different. Talking to older relatives and reading about our ethnic heritage in books such as *Ethnicity and Family Therapy,* Second Edition, by McGoldrick, Giordano, & Pearce (1996) can be very helpful. Those of us fortunate enough to have had our family tree documented by a relative will have a head start in this process.

Questions to ask ourselves include the following:

- How do I respond when asked for my racial, ethnic, or cultural heritage?
- If my family immigrated to this country, when, where, and why? Into what conditions did they arrive?
- Who are the significant "characters" in my family's history?
- How would I describe my attitudes toward family, work, time, independence, competition, material possessions, and sex roles?
- How are these attitudes similar to and different from those of my parents?

Answering these questions thoughtfully will tell us much about our own cultural influences. Discussing them with persons of similar and different ethnic heritage will illustrate that we all have a significant cultural contribution to our history, attitudes, and behaviors. It also is obvious that these influences differ widely by individual.

A third essential element required for cultural competence is consciousness of the dynamics of cultural interaction. A few terms are especially important here. One is *ethnocentrism,* defined as "belief in the superiority of one's own ethnic group" (*American Heritage Dictionary,* 1992, p. 630). Extreme examples of this orientation are cultural genocide, such as the Holocaust of World War II, or the effects of 19th- and 20th-century immigration on the Native American populations of the United States. A second term is *bias,* used as a synonym for *prejudice,* which is defined as "an adverse judgment or opinion formed beforehand without knowledge or examination of the facts" (*American Heritage Dictionary,* 1992, p. 1482). All of us have our biases, whether we are aware of them or not. *Cultural mistrust* describes the sentiment of many people of one culture toward people from another culture. A final term is *white privilege,* which is the concept that European Americans have more power throughout our society, often due simply to the color of their skin. Although white people are largely unaware of this power imbalance, most people of color are very conscious of it.

The concepts defined above are at the heart of the dynamics set into motion when cultures interact. Both European American people and people of color actively participate in of these dynamics. For either group to deny their existence is deceptive and unproductive. Culturally competent individuals and systems recognize these dynamics and continually work at minimizing the negative effects while expanding their own and others' awareness. Such individuals and systems pay attention to how these issues may influence other dynamics of social interaction. For example, Gonzalez-Mena (1997) describes extensive cultural differences around common child-rearing issues such as toilet training, feeding, sleeping, and attachment and separation. Interventionists must be open to hearing what individual parents have to say on these topics and be willing to negotiate or compromise on specific practices when possible.

In Our Practice

Moving to a more outward focus, a fourth element of cultural competence is ongoing expansion of cultural knowledge and resources. Culturally competent individuals and systems make a conscious effort to learn about other cultures. The arts provide many vehicles for this. The dance, theater, films, and literature of cultures other than our own can be simultaneously enjoyable and eye-opening, as can cultivating a taste for a variety of ethnic foods. Having conversations and contact with people of disparate cultures may teach us that we have similarities and differences with everyone. Cultural diversity training is also becoming widely available in many parts of the country.

Although some of these ways of expanding cultural knowledge may be less accessible in rural areas or small towns, reading multicultural fiction, biographies, and poetry is always an option and may be especially instructive. Reference staff in public or college libraries can be a big help in finding this reading material. To avoid stereotyping, it is important to remember that according to the theory of intraethnic variation, there is often more variation within a cultural group than across cultural groups (Campinha-Bacote, 1994).

In addition to expanding our cultural knowledge, it is important to enlarge our cultural resources. This means incorporating artifacts and tools of other cultures into our homes and workplaces. For example, a child care provider may read multicultural children's books to the children, include ethnic dolls and clothing in the dress-up corner, and post photographs of children and families of many cultures throughout the classroom. A family medical practitioner may include ethnic newspapers and magazines in the waiting room, hang the artwork of other cultures on the walls, and refer a chronically ill patient for acupuncture as a complementary treatment. Parents can read multicultural picture books to their young children, provide dolls of different races, choose videos with positive images of other cultures, and encourage contacts with children of other races and religions. Agencies and programs can arrange multicultural potluck dinners and storytelling sessions with their participants and sponsor field trips to ethnic events or exhibits.

The fifth and last element for cultural competence is adaptation to diversity. As Cross et al. (1989) put it, this means working toward a better fit between the needs of minority groups and the services provided. This may mean arranging for an interpreter, offering multicultural experiences and antibias training to our employees, printing notices in alternate languages, expanding our definition of family, recruiting and providing support services to staff members of color, and changing the goals and style of our services. Our energies will be far better spent if we make ongoing efforts to include members of our target populations as we plan and implement these adaptations.

García Coll and Meyer (1993) suggest that clinicians explore several basic questions from their clients' perspective: Is there a problem? Why is there a problem? What can be done? Who should intervene to address the problem? These discussions will open a dialogue between interventionists and parents, clarify issues, and help determine the course of the intervention.

Finally, it is crucial to remember that cultural competence is a developmental process. Cross et al. (1989) discuss a continuum of six possibilities, ranging from cultural destructiveness, to incapacity, to blindness, to precompetence, to competence, to proficiency. Despite where individuals or systems may fall on this continuum, there is always room for positive growth. Although this growth may sometimes be painful and require us to confront our ignorance or guilt, it is essential to our ongoing professional development.

Because much of cultural competence is just good interpersonal skills, we can improve all our human interactions through learning and practicing cultural competence. Campinha-Bacote (1995) suggests that we avoid paralysis by remembering that "we can be so politically correct that we're no earthly good." The good news is that if we are truly committed to empowering families and offering need-driven strategies, we are very apt to become more culturally competent in the process. And when we embrace cultural differences, we will find common goals to meet the universal needs of all children.

MAKING OUR PROGRAMS
AND AGENCIES USER FRIENDLY

In addition to the concepts and approaches discussed earlier in this chapter and book, there are concrete strategies we can use to make our programs and agencies more accessible to a broad range of families. When we create a news release or notice to publicize an event, service, product, or program, public relations professionals tell us to address each of the following questions: "Who, what, when, where, and why?" When we are offering information and services to improve the lives of families of infants and toddlers, we would do well to deal with each of the following: "Who, what, how, and why?"

Relative to the "who" question, there are at least two "whos" to consider. First, whom are we trying to reach? Although we may want to answer this quickly and move on to the next consideration, let's take more time. It can be helpful to use the mindset of a marketing professional. Who is our primary audience? Who else might be interested in/ benefit from our service or product? We can brainstorm all the possibilities, either with colleagues or just with pen and paper or word processor. After listing our audiences, we can analyze the outreach efforts required to reach them. For example, we may consider low-income single parents to be a high priority audience, but realize that special and sustained "marketing" strategies may be required to gain their participation.

The second "who" to think about concerns the relationship building that is at the heart of any service provision. In Chapter 3, we discussed the concept of people's working models, that is, what they have come to expect of other people based on their past social experiences. We need to think about the possible working models of our target audiences. In some cases, it may be important to contradict these expectations. If a young mother's working model of others, based on previous experience, is that they are undependable and uncaring, service providers will need to persist patiently until she identifies them as dependable and caring. These qualities underpin the process of relationship building, and until a positive relationship is established between provider and participant, service provision is likely to be unproductive.

In considering the "what," the content of our program or service must be well thought out and clearly presented. In earlier sections of this chapter and book, we discuss what "well thought out" means. We'll focus here on clear presentation. As mentioned above, public relations professionals suggest any presentation include the "who, what, when, where, and why" of our program, event, or service. Any printed material should include these elements, plus a "to register" or "for further information" category with a telephone number or address. We should aim for a simple reading level and avoid using jargon. With word processors widely available, it is quite simple to make printed materials attractive, and there is no longer any excuse for them to be handwritten or unappealing. Even if our agency or program does not have a word processor, it is worth the extra time and expense to find someone to make our material pleasing to the eye. The whole point of printed information is to get people to read it. They are far more likely to do so if it is simply written and attractively presented.

In addition to having eye appeal, information should also be psychologically appealing. This means that we consider what might be of most interest or utility to our audience when we plan our topics or write our handouts and informational pieces. For example, parents of newborns might be interested in breast- and/or bottlefeeding, parents of 6-month-olds in childproofing their home for safety, and parents of toddlers in handling temper tantrums. What is the most essential information on each of these subjects? For tip sheets, what lead-in heading or sentence will pull these readers in? What closing will wrap the information up most succinctly?

Regarding the "how" of making our agencies user friendly, we need to focus on logistics for our participants. Foremost among these are transportation, scheduling, cost, and location. Just as any facility serving the public considers how it will provide convenient free or low-cost parking, it also needs to consider its accessibility to users of public transportation. In areas without public transportation, some families will need assistance with transportation if they are to participate in program offerings. For most families with small children who do not have access to a reliable vehicle, getting to and from appointments, grocery shopping, employment, and other destinations for ongoing necessities can consume inordinate amounts of time and become a logistical nightmare. This issue is compounded in climates with harsh weather and in sparsely populated rural areas. Organizations need to appraise carefully the transportation needs of all families they intend to serve. Strategies such as car pooling, public transportation or taxi vouchers, vans, swapping transportation help for technical assistance with another agency, and locating with or near other essential services are all possible methods to address this issue.

Scheduling of offerings needs to be convenient for families. Employed parents may appreciate a parent education discussion group that meets weekly with a light meal at 5:30 P.M. at their child's care center. If we want to reach a variety of parents, evening and weekend scheduling must be added to morning and afternoon times. We may want to avoid scheduling toddler parent group events in the early afternoon when toddlers are likely to be napping. This same time may be fine for parents of newborns whose children have not yet developed anything resembling regular sleep habits. It may be helpful to limit the length of any parent group meetings to 2 hours or less if infants and toddlers are also attending, as that's about how long small ones can last before requiring feeding, diapering, or napping from a familiar caregiver.

Cost of program offerings depends on whom we are trying to reach. When working with low-income families, services should be at low or no cost to participants. Sliding fee scales may work well when we are serving a cross-section of parents by income level. These should be simple and based on an honor system on the part of families, without requiring tax returns or other evidence of income level. For suggested income categories, one source is the annually updated federal free and reduced lunch guidelines used by public schools. First-time attendance and special family events can be offered free of charge to help draw in families. For families who cannot afford even low program fees, the agency can offer "scholarships" on request, no questions asked.

Location of program services is very important, a fact that is obvious to any business owner or real estate agent. Convenience is very important to all families in today's fast-paced society. Increasingly across the country, communities are creating family centers designed to respond to local needs. A variety of agencies will often work together to offer a range of services to a broad number of families within one convenient location. The menu of offerings often includes health care; parent support groups; information and referral; literacy classes; used clothing exchanges; toy libraries; Women, Infant, and Children (WIC) food programs; counseling; housing assistance; and/or whatever services are most needed in that particular community.

The facility needs to be clean, attractive, and welcoming to infants, toddlers, young children, and parents. Family centers are located in diverse places such as churches, schools, libraries, shopping centers, clinics, apartment complexes, and so forth. Whether services are offered in a family center or independent agency, locating them near bus or subway lines in cities, and main roads in small-town or rural areas, will make them more conducive to family participation.

As for the "why," we must continually reassess the need for our information and services so as to be certain that there is a demand for them. Education, health, and social service professionals can fall too easily into a "but we've always done it this way" mentality. This limited approach stunts creativity and diminishes individualization for the broad variety of client families. Just as contemporary middle- and upper-income families may purchase errand-running and meal preparation services, in addition to or instead of more traditional housecleaning and child care services, so may lower-income families have altered and/or expanding public assistance requirements. With times rapidly changing, what may have been appropriate support for families 10 years ago may no longer be suitable. Utilizing market research techniques, such as consumer satisfaction surveys or focus groups, can help us identify why we do what we do and how we can make it better and more useful for families.

Offering incentives for participation will also tangibly address the "why" for families. Meals or refreshments are almost always appreciated by busy parents and children of all income levels and cultural backgrounds. The foods selected can serve an educational purpose as well, with healthy selections presented simply and appealingly and/or ethnic foods demonstrating the program's respect for diverse cultures. Other incentives include libraries of books and toys, inclusive family holiday celebrations, and certificates of participation. Helping families secure other needed services and items such as safe housing or warm winter clothing, although these may not be standard program offerings, serves as an incentive to program participation. Establishing a barter network among families and with program staff may reduce dollar expenses. For example, one parent can cook a meal for another in exchange for occasional child care, parents and staff members can contribute to a clothing and children's toy exchange in a family center, or parents can help build a loft area in a child care center in exchange for a portion of tuition. In addition to its utility, bartering also illustrates reciprocity and mutual respect, values that enrich human life.

THE ROLE OF THE DOMINANT CULTURE

An important macrosystem influence on a family is the culture surrounding it, both its immediate culture and ethnicity, and the larger or dominant culture. The critical role of the larger culture in placing serious stressors on families must be recognized and acknowledged. For example, Leach (1994) identifies individualism and competition as the overall "social ethos" of our Western society. She notes that these values are not conducive to effective parenting and productive family life, which require sharing and cooperation. Garbarino (1995a) argues that children today are growing up in a socially toxic environment. He cites the prevalence of violence in our communities and in the media, the proliferation of guns and assault weapons among adolescents, the presence of AIDS, high divorce rates, poverty and other economic pressures, the expanding variety and accessibility of illegal drugs, and the reduction of adult time spent interacting with and supervising children and adolescents. This socially toxic environment increases the demands on parents to be more vigilant caregivers and on schools to produce competent children.

Those of us who are earning an adequate income and living in two-parent households in reasonably safe neighborhoods know that contemporary family life is stressful. Those of us who are unemployed or employed at low-wage jobs and living alone with our children are more likely to live in dangerous neighborhoods and struggle daily to meet our family's most basic needs.

Garbarino (1995a) discusses how the monetarization of our industrial economy has devalued activities that do not earn wages. Families are requiring more and more income to meet basic needs, and what they define as basic needs is expanding steadily as a result of our profit-driven consumer economy. For example, paper diapers are now considered by many, if not most, parents to be a necessity, although they cost considerably more than cloth diapers. Because of a lack of universally accessible systems for health care, child care, housing, and other basic human needs, low income is a better predictor of child development problems in the United States than in other countries (Garbarino, 1995a).

One of the factors contributing to a socially toxic environment regardless of a family's income level is the presence of television in more than 98% of American homes. The average preschooler watches 28 hours per week, and older children watch on average 23.5 hours per week (Nielsen Media Research, 1993). Researchers have documented the effects of television violence on children, and these effects are very real and quite negative (Paik & Comstock, 1994). They include increased aggression and desensitization, so that more and more violence is required to elicit an emotional response. In addition, commonsense tells us that the violence, sexism, racism, and rampant consumerism of most of private television and its incessant commercial interruptions do not promote the kind of values that most parents hold dear. The addition of computers to an expanding number of contemporary homes compounds children's potential exposure to violence and inappropriate sexual content through computer games and Internet sites.

Clearly, a new charge has been added to the role of parents as socialization agents for their children in the late 20th century and beyond. In the past, family life was largely shaped by the guidance of community and culture. Today, due in large part to the high mobility of American families, many parents do not have friends or family members in the communities where they live. To find this sense of community, parents must consciously work at building supportive relationships within their neighborhoods, places of worship, and/or workplaces. Familial isolation, combined with the explosion of new technology and the pressure of commercial values, may result in community and culture serving as sources of stress rather than coherent structure or support.

In order to create or preserve a healthy family life, parents must be *intentional* about shaping the type of life they want within and around their families (Doherty, 1997). This implies limiting the time demands of outside activities on family members and carefully monitoring the quantity and quality of technology use within households. It also means being more intentional about structuring the routines of daily family living. As interventionists, we can support families as they attempt to meet these new challenges.

SUMMARY

As the 20th century draws to a close and we enter a new millennium, it is obvious that our daily lives have been changing dramatically and swiftly. We've moved from a largely agrarian economy to an industrial economy to what many are calling a technological economy. These massive changes have had profound effects on family life over time. Some of these effects are positive, but many are negative and largely unintended by-products of exploding technology and the increasingly fast pace of daily life. Community and culture, which have been the primary sources of structure and support for families, may now be sources of stress. Many of the strategies we discuss in this chapter will help to rebuild more intentional communities and family-friendly culture.

These strategies are grounded in a new view of power as a capacity to bring about positive change, as an entity that expands the more it is shared, and as a system in which no participant is powerless. If as interventionists we view our role not as service providers *for* families, but as partners and facilitators *with* families, helping them to recognize and expand their available resources, we can be far more effective than we have been in the past. Despite our best efforts, however, there are many barriers to families using resources. We offer specific and practical ideas for working with families to assess their resources for support and overcome common barriers to using these resources.

Home visiting and parent support groups are important vehicles for strengthening family support networks, and we consider major components and issues inherent in their implementation. Because cultural competence is integral to working respectfully and productively with diverse families, we look at creative techniques to expand our understanding and skills in this area. To paraphrase Garbarino (1995b), we believe that every culture has something to teach, and every culture has something to learn. This concept also applies to every parent and to every interventionist and is embedded in the strategies we suggest throughout this chapter.

CONCLUSION

Working with infants and toddlers and their families can be challenging, exhausting, unpredictable, and frustrating. It is also interesting, energizing, fascinating, and incredibly rewarding. The unprecedented media attention devoted to new developments in neuroscience presents interventionists with both a new challenge and new opportunity. The challenge includes clarifying the now-or-never emphasis on maximizing infant brain development through stimulation, reading, and even educational videos designed and marketed specifically for babies. Many of these strategies are antithetical to the way that infants and toddlers learn best, that is, by interacting with the people and objects in their environment, at their own pace and in their own style.

These prescriptive approaches also trivialize the importance of individualization and of sensitivity to the wide differences in infant temperament from birth on. Some babies love to be read to from a few months of age, whereas others will not sit still for even the most enticing picture book until they are 3 or older. Contemporary parents of infants and toddlers do not need any more unnecessary "shoulds" in their busy lives.

Parents do need support and information to assist them in understanding and managing their child's behaviors and responding sensitively to his or her communication cues and signals. Perhaps most important in our hurried world, parents and families need support and encouragement to pay attention to and appreciate the amazing growth and development of their own children.

The birth of every baby is and always has been a miracle. In each case, it offers new potential for a human being to enrich and enhance the course of the future and of history. So in essence, our most important new opportunity as we work with families of infants and toddlers underscores one of our long-held goals in the field of early intervention. We hope to promote the capacity of each new human person to fulfill his or her intellectual, social, emotional, and physical potential in a rapidly changing world that needs all the potential it can get.

REFERENCES

American heritage dictionary of the English language (3rd ed.). (1992). Boston, MA: Houghton Mifflin.

Bronfenbrenner, U. (1979). *The ecology of human development: Experiments by nature and design.* Cambridge, MA: Harvard University Press.

Bronfenbrenner, U. (1987). Foreword. In S. L. Kagan, D. R. Powell, B. Weissbourd, & E. F. Zigler (Eds.), *America's family support programs: Perspectives and prospects* (pp. xi–xvii). New Haven: Yale University Press.

Campinha-Bacote, J. (1994). *The process of cultural competence in health care: A culturally competent model of care* (2nd ed.). Wyoming, OH: Transcultural C.A.R.E. Associates.

Campinha-Bacote, J. (1995, November). *Culturally competent services: What are they?* Paper presented at the Fourth Annual Symposium of St. David's School for Child Development and Family Services, Minneapolis.

Carter, N. (1995). *Parenting education in the United States: An investigative report.* Philadelphia: Pew Charitable Trusts.

Cooke, B. (1992). *Changing times, changing families: Minnesota early childhood family education parent outcome interview study.* St. Paul: Minnesota Department of Children, Families, and Learning.

Cross, T. L., Bazron, B. J., Dennis, K. W., & Isaacs, M. R. (1989, March). *Towards a culturally competent system of care: A monograph on effective services for minority children who are severely emotionally disturbed.* Washington, DC: Georgetown University Child Development Center, CASSP Technical Assistance Center.

Curran, D. (1983). *Traits of a healthy family.* Minneapolis: Winston Press.

Doherty, W. J. (1997). *The intentional family: How to build family ties in our modern world.* Reading, MA: Addison-Wesley.

Dunst, C. J., & Trivette, C. M. (1990). Assessment of social support in early intervention programs. In S. J. Meisels & J. P. Shonkoff (Eds.), *Handbook of early childhood intervention* (pp. 326–349). New York: Cambridge University Press.

Dunst, C. J., Trivette, C. M., & Deal, A. G. (1988). *Enabling and empowering families: Principles and guidelines for practice.* Cambridge, MA: Brookline Books.

Dunst, C. J., Trivette, C. M., & Deal, A. G. (Eds.). (1994). *Supporting and strengthening families: Vol. 1. Methods, strategies, and practices.* Cambridge, MA: Brookline Books.

Erickson, M. F., & Simon, J. (1999). *Steps toward effective, enjoyable parenting: Facilitators' guide.* Minneapolis: Irving B. Harris Training Center for Infant and Toddler Development, University of Minnesota.

Garbarino, J. (1995a). *Raising children in a socially toxic environment.* San Francisco: Jossey-Bass.

Garbarino, J. (1995b, May). *Raising children in a socially toxic environment.* Paper presented at the Early Childhood Family Education Coordinators Conference, Minneapolis.

García Coll, C. T., & Meyer, E. C. (1993). The sociocultural context of infant development. In C. H. Zeanah, Jr. (Ed.), *Handbook of infant mental health* (pp. 56–69). New York: Guilford Press.

Gonzalez-Mena, J. (1997). *Multicultural issues in child care.* Mountain View, CA: Mayfield.

Hobbs, N., Dokecki, P. R., Hoover-Dempsey, K. V., Moroney, R. M., Shayne, M. W., & Weeks, K. H. (1984). *Strengthening families.* San Francisco: Jossey-Bass.

Katz, R. (1984). Empowerment and synergy: Expanding the community's healing process. In J. Rappaport, C. Swift, & R. Hess (Eds.), *Studies in empowerment: Steps toward understanding and action* (pp. 201–226). New York: Haworth Press.

Klass, C. S. (1996). *Home visiting: Promoting healthy parent and child development.* Baltimore: Brookes.

Lappe, F. M., & DuBois, P. M. (1994). *The quickening of America: Rebuilding our nation, remaking our lives.* San Francisco: Jossey-Bass.

Leach, P. (1994). *Children first: What our society must do—and is not doing— for our children today.* New York: Knopf.

Lynch, E. W., & Hanson, M. J. (1992). *Developing cross-cultural competence: A guide for working with young children and their families.* Baltimore: Brookes.

McGoldrick, M., Giordano, J., & Pearce, J. K. (Eds.). (1996). *Ethnicity and family therapy* (2nd ed.). New York: Guilford Press.

McKnight, J. (1989, April). *Beyond community services.* Unpublished manuscript, Center for Urban Affairs and Policy Research, Northwestern University, Evanston, IL.

Morgaine, C. B. (1988). *Process parenting: Breaking the addictive cycle.* St. Paul: Minnesota Department of Human Services.

Nielsen Media Research. (1993). *1992–93 report on television.* New York: Author.

Olds, D. L., Henderson, C. R., Jr., Tatelbaum, R., & Chamberlin, R. (1988). Improving the life-course development of socially disadvantaged mothers: A randomized trial of nurse home visitation. *American Journal of Public Health, 78,* 1436–1445.

Paik, H., & Comstock, G. (1994). The effects of televised violence on antisocial behavior: A meta-analysis. *Communication Research, 21,* 516–546.

Pilusuk, M., & Parks, S. H. (1986). *The healing web: Social networks and human survival.* Hanover, NH: University Press of New England.

Pooley, L. E. (Ed.). (1994). *Learning to be partners: An introductory training program for family support staff.* Chicago: Family Resource Coalition.

Powell, D. R. (1995, September). *Teaching parenting and basic skills to parents: What we know.* Paper presented at Research Design Symposium on Family Literacy, U.S. Department of Education, Office of Educational Research and Improvement, Washington, DC.

Wasik, B. H., Bryant, D. M., & Lyons, C. M. (1990). *Home visiting: Procedures for helping families.* Newbury Park, CA: Sage.

Weiss, H. B. (1993). Home visits: Necessary but not sufficient. In *Home visiting: Vol. 3 No. 3. The future of children* (pp. 113–128). Los Altos, CA: David and Lucile Packard Foundation.

Weissbourd, B. (1987). A brief history of family support programs. In S. L. Kagan, D. R. Powell, B. Weissbourd, & E. F. Zigler (Eds.), *America's family support programs: Perspectives and prospects* (pp. 38–56). New Haven: Yale University Press.

APPENDIX

Resource Bibliography

BOOKS AND CURRICULUM/TRAINING RESOURCES

Abidin, Richard. (1996). *Early childhood parenting skills.* Odessa, FL: Psychological Assessment Resources.

Using a thoughtfully eclectic approach, Richard Abidin has written a parent education manual that draws on the wisdom of four psychological schools of thought: self-concept theory, relationship and humanistic communications, behavioral principles, and cognitive psychology. Abidin's focus is not to suggest a "right way" to parent, but rather to support parents as they develop the "insight and skills necessary to reach their own parenting goals" (p. vi). The 340-page manual for professionals and the accompanying 139-page workbook for parents encompass information gleaned from research literature, interviews with 50 child development professionals, and discussions with hundreds of parents. Although the manual is highly structured with specific suggestions for group activities, it is designed for flexible use in a variety of settings. The manual contains background information on important issues including program evaluation; 19 education sessions that address child development, parent–child relationships, and managing parents' feelings; and five single-session lectures/ workshops for community presentations. One caution: Program activities and home practice exercises have a heavy emphasis on reading and writing, with a classroom type of style that will not be appropriate for all parents.

Alexander, Shoshana. (1994). *In praise of single parents: Mothers and fathers embracing the challenge.* Boston: Houghton Mifflin.

In much of the current debate about welfare reform, the single-parent family is cited as the root of many of society's ills. For single-parent families, this vilification is hardly helpful and often profoundly discouraging. Under the best of circumstances, parenting is a difficult and challenging endeavor. Yet each single-parent family has its unique strengths and challenges, as does each two-parent family. Shoshana Alexander, a single parent herself, has written a thoughtful and encouraging book about the unique strengths and challenges of single parenting. Much more than a catalog of helpful tips, *In Praise of Single Parents* examines issues such as embracing the challenge of single parenting whether one has become one by chance or by choice, perfection and guilt, nurturing oneself, finances, child care, discipline, dating, dealing with the absent parent, and extending the family. This book is positive and inspiring, as well as practical.

Bailey, Pam, Cryer, Debby, Harms, Thelma, Osborne, Sheri, & Kniest, Barbara A. (1996). *Active learning for children with disabilities: A manual for use with the Active Learning Series.* Menlo Park, CA: Addison-Wesley.

Designed for use with the Active Learning Series (see Cryer, Harms, & Bourland below), this manual provides information on activities for infants, toddlers, and preschoolers with disabilities. It points out that interventionists and caregivers do not need to alter drastically the way they do things when a child with a disability enters the program. Most of the time, only three steps are necessary: Plan each day's activities to include those children with disabilities, making changes as needed; arrange the setting so that children with disabilities can be with other children and take part in all activities; and change some materials and activities so that children with disabilities can use them. This manual provides solid, practical information for implementing these three steps.

Beal, Anne, Villarosa, Linda, & Abner, Allison. (1999). *The black parenting book.* New York: Broadway Books.

This book is an excellent addition to the literature for parents of children from birth to age 5 and parent educators. Written by a pediatrician and two journalists, all African American mothers of young children, *The Black Parenting Book* uses clear understandable language, offers a good menu of suggestions rather than prescriptions for common parenting issues, and is culturally specific while consistent with the findings of current child development research. It combines sound and comprehensive information with specific practical advice, including hair and skin care. Each of the 15 chapters concludes with a helpful resource list.

Belsky, Jay, & Nezworski, Teresa (Eds.). (1987). *Clinical implications of attachment.* Hillsdale, NJ: Erlbaum.

This 440-page volume presents a comprehensive discussion of attachment issues, research on antecedents and consequences of different patterns of attachment, and clinical applications of attachment theory and research. It is a significant effort toward bridging the gap between research and practice and is a good resource for practitioners interested in this important topic.

Blau, Melinda. (1993). *Families apart: Ten keys to successful co-parenting.* New York: Berkley.

This book is a very helpful tool for parents, parent educators, and other interventionists who work with divorced parents. The author makes the point that she is not promoting the benefits of divorce, but is proposing better ways to parent children after the decision to divorce. The central goal of this is to minimize the negative effects of divorce on children and promote their healthy development after divorce. Her chapter titles reflect her 10 strategies: heal yourself after divorce, act maturely, listen to your children, respect each other as parents, divide parenting time, accept each other's differences, communicate about (and with) the children, step outside traditional gender roles, anticipate and accept change, and know that co-parenting is forever.

Brazelton, T. Berry. (1992). *Touchpoints: Your child's emotional and behavioral development.* Reading, MA: Addison-Wesley.

Probably America's best-known pediatrician and a prolific writer, T. Berry Brazelton distills in this book his 40 years of pediatric experience into what he calls a "map" of infancy and early childhood development. He defines "touchpoints" as those universal, predictable periods that occur just before a surge of rapid growth in any area of development, when a child's behavior falls apart for a short time. He feels that these touchpoints are valuable windows through which parents can view the incredible energy that fuels a child's desire for learning. They also illuminate a child's strengths, weaknesses, and temperamental tendencies and are a unique opportunity to understand the child better as an individual. The book is divided into three sections, which define the touchpoints from pregnancy through 3 years of age; discuss common child-rearing issues that emerge during this period; and address the influences of parents, grandparents, caregivers, and others on child development. An excellent and comprehensive resource, this book will be helpful to parents and should be required on the bookshelves of all physicians, other health professionals, social workers, child care providers, parent educators, and others who work with very young children and their families.

Brazelton, T. Berry, & Cramer, Bertrand G. (1990). *The earliest relationship: Parents, infants, and the drama of early attachment.* Reading, MA: Addison-Wesley.

Cowritten by well-known pediatrician T. Berry Brazelton and Bertrand Cramer, a pioneering infant psychiatrist specializing in mother–infant psychotherapy, this work is an interesting blend of the two perspectives. According to the authors, the book is based on two assumptions: that the parent–infant pair must be cared for as a unit and the approach must be trandisciplinary (inclusive of pediatrics, psychiatry, psychology, nursing, social work, and education). Focusing on the growth of parent–child attachment, which is rooted in long-past experiences and develops further during pregnancy through the early years of life, the book stresses the reciprocity of the parent–child relationship through combining developmental observation and analytic insight. It includes discussion of the father's role in this process and stresses the active participation of the newborn and infant. It concludes with nine case studies that illustrate this complementary approach to assessing infants through deeper understanding of their relationships with their primary caregivers. Its thoughtful discussion of Selma Fraiberg's concept of "ghosts in the nursery" examines the influence of families of origin on parenting. *The Earliest Relationship* is an engrossing description of the psychoanalytic perspective on parent–child attachment.

Bredekamp, Sue, & Copple, Carol. (Eds.). (1997). *Developmentally appropriate practice in early childhood programs* (rev. ed.). Washington, DC: National Association for the Education of Young Children.

These criteria were initially developed in response to the need for a clearer definition of developmentally appropriate practice to implement the National Association for the Education of Young Children (NAEYC) accreditation system for early childhood programs. The guidelines represent the consensus of hundreds of early childhood professionals, with the revised edition incorporating new research and current best practice in the early childhood field. The book begins with a discussion of principles of child development and learning. It continues with a definition of "developmentally appropriate" and overall guidelines for teacher decision making. It then proceeds with a discussion of typical development for infants and toddlers, for 3- through 5-year-olds, and for 6- through 8-year-olds. In each age-specific section, the text is followed by clearly formatted examples of appropriate and inappropriate practice. This book is an essential tool for teachers, administrators, and policymakers concerned with the quality of early childhood programs.

Bromwich, Rose. (1997). *Working with families and their infants at risk: A perspective after 20 years of experience.* Austin, TX: PRO-ED.

Continuing her premise that enhancing parent–infant interaction is a primary strategy for early interventionists, Rose Bromwich has updated and expanded her 1981 book, which was focused on infants at risk for physically or mentally disabling conditions. She now includes discussion of adolescent mothers, as well as parents who are mentally ill, mentally retarded, chemically dependent, or have other risk factors for healthy parenting. The most useful information appears in Chapters 5 and 6, most of which were featured in her earlier book. These chapters describe the intervention strategies used by Bromwich and her colleagues and provide specific and detailed responses to a variety of problems in social–affective, cognitive–motivational, language, and motor areas of infant development.

Brown, Wesley S., Thurman, Kenneth, & Pearl, Lynda. (Eds.). (1993). *Family-centered early intervention with infants and toddlers: Innovative cross-disciplinary approaches.* Baltimore: Brookes.

As its title indicates, this book is a collection of topical chapters addressing early intervention through cross-disciplinary lenses. It begins with a thorough discussion of the legislative context for early intervention, focusing especially on the Part H program of Public Law 99-457. Subsequent chapters focus on defining eligibility, assessment and evaluation, collaboration and service coordination, curricula, intervention in the neonatal intensive care unit, and follow-up of at-risk infants. A thoughtful review follows of the services and roles provided by a wide variety of early intervention professionals such as physicians, physical therapists, early childhood special educators, and so forth. Concluding chapters of the book examine program evaluation and continuing issues in early intervention. This publication is a good resource for preservice and in-service training of all professionals who work with infants and toddlers with disabilities.

Bryant, Donna M., & Graham, Mimi A. (Eds.). (1993). *Implementing early intervention: From research to effective practice.* New York: Guilford Press.

Designed as a reference for professionals implementing the mandate of Public Law 99-457 and Part H, this book is a comprehensive collection of writing by leading experts on eligibility and assessment, family-centered and effective intervention practices, administration, and public policy. It provides the context for services, detailed information about specific services, and suggestions for state and federal policy development for early intervention.

Chen, Milton. (1994). *The smart parent's guide to kids' TV.* San Francisco: KQED Books.

The author, a long-time researcher and educator for public television in San Francisco, provides refreshingly simple and practical strategies for parents who want to maximize the positive and minimize the negative potential of television. After documenting the enormous presence television has in the average American home and the clear link between television violence and aggressive behavior, Chen offers commonsense advice on how to use television as a learning tool, rather than banning it all together. As Joan Ganz Cooney, originator of *Sesame Street,* states in the book's preface, "This book should be packaged with every new TV and VCR sold to a parent, just as a sample of detergent comes with a washing machine."

Comer, James, & Poussaint, Alvin. (1992). *Raising black children.* New York: Penguin Books USA.

A revision of the 1975 book *Black Child Care,* this book was written out of the black awareness movement of the 1970s. As the authors state, "Growing up black in America, where most policy-making and attitudes are influenced and controlled by whites who are often antagonistic or indifferent to the needs of blacks, poses many special problems for black parents and their children." In addition to issues of race, black parents must deal with the normal developmental challenges that all children present. Written in an easily readable question-and-answer format, *Raising Black Children* begins with an overview of America and the black child and proceeds in a straightforward, no-nonsense style through all the developmental stages of childhood, from infancy through adolescence. It spends three chapters on the often-overlooked school-age years, asserting that these are critical years for cognitive, social, and emotional growth. This book is an excellent resource for black parents and anyone who works with black children.

Cramer, Lina. (1991). *Parent time curriculum guide: A learning activities guide for the PACE family literacy program.* Chicago: Family Resource Coalition.

Packaged for ready insertion into a 3-ring binder, this curriculum is an excellent resource for parent educators and support group facilitators. It begins with a useful overview of the group facilitation process and proceeds to creative and participatory learning activities structured around parents in their roles as persons, parents, students, family members, community members, and workers. Well-organized and attractive, the guide also includes reproducible handouts for parents.

Cryer, Debby, Harms, Thelma, & Bourland, Beth. (1987 and 1988). Addison-Wesley Active Learning Series: *Active learning for infants, Active learning for ones,* and *Active learning for twos.* Menlo Park, CA: Addison-Wesley.

Produced by child care professionals from the Frank Porter Graham Child Development Center at the University of North Carolina in Chapel Hill, this series is a collection of separate activity books for infants, and 1-, 2-, and 3-year-olds. Each book begins with a helpful planning guide and has four activity sections: activities for listening and talking, activities for physical development, creative activities, and activities for learning from the surrounding world. The activities are clearly presented and graphically coded for age level, outdoor or indoor activity, typical time the activity takes, and the number of babies one could include in the activity (helpful for group care providers). These books are a comprehensive curriculum resource for child care providers and also can be used by parents and parent educators.

Curran, Delores. (1989). *Working with parents: Delores Curran's guide to successful parent groups.* Circle Pines, MN: American Guidance Service.

In order to be effective, infant and toddler service providers must work with the parents of their young clients. Writing for professionals such as educators, nurses, clergy, psychologists, or social workers, the author encourages all of these people also to define themselves proudly as parent educators. *Working with Parents* provides a practical approach to the issues and specifics of working with parents individually and in groups. Beginning by examining some traditional assumptions many professionals have about working with parents, the book discusses good needs-assessment and listening techniques, how to empower parents, effective lecture tips, dealing with "problem" parents, parent group facilitation, effective one-on-one conferences, and career possibilities in parent education. It concludes with a resource section and several handouts and surveys that may be reproduced for use in parent education settings.

Davis, Laura, & Keyser, Janis. (1997). *Becoming the parent you want to be: A sourcebook of strategies for the first five years.* New York: Broadway Books.

Written by the author of *The Courage to Heal* (a resource for incest survivors) and by a long-time parent educator, this book is an exceptional addition to the literature for parents and for parent educators. Comprehensive and loaded with practical suggestions, it focuses on the kind of thoughtful, purposeful parenting that tends to produce thoughtful, competent children. The book begins with a framework of nine principles for parenting and follows with sections on children's feelings, children's bodies, difficult behavior, social learning and play, and family relationships. Whether discussing sleep issues, feeding, separation, biting, or any other relevant topic, the authors offer multiple strategies without being prescriptive or contradictory, always encouraging parents to try new ideas and learn from their mistakes.

Doherty, William J. (1997). *The intentional family: How to build family ties in our modern world.* Reading, MA: Addison-Wesley.

William Doherty, an experienced family therapist and father of two, argues that today's families must work intentionally at maintaining and building family ties. Without this effort, contemporary family life loses its energy and coherence, conspired against by the lack of societal support for family life, time pressures, and electronic technology within our homes. The author suggests two main strategies to strengthen family life. The first is to make better use of the time we already spend on family activities, such as meals, bedtimes, morning routines, and so forth. The second strategy is to reclaim time from activities that take more than their fair share, such as television and other home technology. His book offers specific and practical suggestions for making enjoyable rituals out of the stuff of daily life. Holidays, birthdays, weddings, and funerals are also included as fertile ground for fresh and flexible rituals. Concluding with special considerations for single parents and remarried families, this book is a treasure chest, both for newly formed families and for all families seeking to revitalize their relationships.

Dunst, Carl, Trivette, Carol, & Deal, Angela. (1988). *Enabling and empowering families: Principles and guidelines for practice.* Cambridge, MA: Brookline Books.

One of the earlier books to promote the empowerment approach to working with families of special needs and at-risk children, this book is a classic in its field. The book evolved from 7 years of research and clinical work at the Family, Infant, and Preschool Program in Morganton, North Carolina. Its eight chapters comprehensively cover topics related to family functioning and a family systems approach to assessment and intervention. Its appendices consist of a variety of instruments designed for assessing family strengths and needs, and planning for intervention. A separate, full-sized packet of the scales reprinted in the book is available from the publisher.

Dunst, Carl, Trivette, Carol, & Deal, Angela. (1994). *Supporting and strengthening families: Vol. 1. Methods, strategies, and practices.* Cambridge, MA: Brookline Books.

Expanding on the themes introduced in their 1988 book *Enabling and Empowering Families,* Dunst and colleagues introduce two new themes in their most recent book. They argue that traditional human services models and practices are not effective in working with families and suggest that practitioners use the guiding principles and practices that underpin family support programs. (See Chapter 5, this volume, for a discussion of these guiding principles.) Secondly, in an attempt to diffuse the long-standing human service controversy between prioritizing either treatment or prevention services, Dunst et al. propose that we enhance and *promote* the competencies and capabilities of all people. Although when read straight through the book is rather repetitive, it is a storehouse of concrete suggestions, as its title suggests, for supporting and strengthening families.

Epstein, Ann, Larner, Mary, & Halpern, Robert. (1995). *A guide to developing community-based family support programs.* Ypsilanti, MI: High/Scope Press.

This guide was created for program developers and administrators considering, planning, or refining family support programs. The authors are veterans of two demonstration efforts—Child Survival/Fair Start and the High/Scope Parent-to-Parent Project. Very comprehensive in scope, the guide includes discussion of a definition and brief history of family support programs; identifying the client population; setting program goals and objectives; program format options, both home and center based; timing and duration of services; curriculum options; staffing structure; staff recruitment, development, and supervision; family recruitment; establishing ties with families; coordinating with other agencies; and evaluating the program.

Erickson, Martha Farrell, & Simon, Jill. (1999). *Steps toward effective, enjoyable parenting: Facilitators' guide.* Minneapolis: Irving B. Harris Training Center for Infant and Toddler Development, University of Minnesota.

Based on attachment theory and research, and informed by findings from evaluations of the STEEP program, this manual is written for professionals and paraprofessionals who work with parents from pregnancy through the first 2 years of a child's life. Opening sections describe the research background for the program and principles for effective home visiting and group work with new parents who are considered high risk because of current circumstances or life history. Subsequent sections, organized chronologically by child's age, provide information on infant/toddler development, parenting issues that are common during those stages, and suggested activities both for group sessions and individual home visits. Throughout, the emphasis is on relationships and the power of people to work together to move beyond old patterns that undermine competence and well-being. Although the manual is specific to the STEEP model, the information can be adapted easily to any program that works with parents and young children.

Fenichel, Emily. (1992). *Learning through supervision and mentorship to support the development of infants, toddlers, and their families: A source book.* Washington, DC: Zero to Three: National Center for Infants, Toddlers, and Families.

This book is a product of a 1991–1992 project that convened a multidisciplinary work group of 10 professionals skilled in the training for and practice of infant and toddler development. Its goals were to examine supervision and mentoring as crucial elements in practitioner training and to suggest strategies for incorporating these elements into training and practice institutions and systems. The work group identified three essential features of effective supervision and mentoring: reflection, collaboration, and regularity. After discussing these features and their common obstacles, the following three sections look at supervision and mentoring of students, supervision and mentoring of practitioners, and issues for supervisors and program directors. A welcome addition to a somewhat uncharted area of supervision, this book will help supervisors and managers better guide the development of the students and practitioners with whom they work. (Also available as part of a video training package; see Gilkerson et al. below)

Ferguson, Gloria. (1995). *Tools for mother–baby interventions.* St. Paul, MN: Health Start.

Building on the University of Minnesota's STEEP program, these rich curriculum resources were developed by staff of several Health Start projects serving Ramsey County, Minnesota, and surrounding areas. Health Start is a private, nonprofit organization that offers "parent education and support to women identified as at high risk for child abuse and neglect due to social isolation, unmet personal needs, high levels of life stress, poor social histories, and lack of knowledge of child care and development." The tools are formatted for easy copying and use and are organized by the following categories: avoiding violence, new parent, discipline, growing child, journals, mother focused, miscellaneous, and self-care. Practical, creative, and thoughtful, these exercises and handouts are highly recommended for interventionists from all disciplines to use in parent discussion groups. The materials come ready for insertion into a three-ring binder and are available for $10 (includes postage and handling) from Health Start, 590 Park Street, Suite 208, St. Paul, MN, 55103.

Fontanel, Beatrice, & d'Harcourt, Claire. (1998). *Babies celebrated*. New York: Abrams.

This visually stunning book is a collection of beautiful color photographs with brief descriptive text on babies in tribal societies around the world. The authors interviewed a team of nearly 20 ethnologists (scientists who analyze and compare human cultures), as well as reviewing their photographs and research. Out of this effort emerged this intriguing look at how babies in tribal societies are washed and massaged, protected and clothed, stowed and carried, rocked and comforted, and cared for by parents and other family and community members. A respectful and reflective introduction by a research director sets the stage for this eye-opening, thought-provoking book.

Fraiberg, Louis. (Ed.). (1987). *Selected writings of Selma Fraiberg*. Columbus: Ohio State University Press.

Selma Fraiberg was a pioneer in the infant mental health movement, and her work continues to have a profound influence on early intervention. Edited by her husband following her death, this large volume presents 29 of Fraiberg's most significant papers, including the eloquent "Ghosts in the Nursery," which describes therapeutic strategies for helping parents break free of their own history of abuse and move toward healthy interaction with their children. Fraiberg's writings about her research and clinical work with blind babies and their parents will be of particular interest to professionals who work with families of infants with disabilities.

Garbarino, James. (1992). *Children and families in the social environment* (2nd ed.). Hawthorne, NY: Aldine de Gruyter.

This is the second edition of a book used in many college-level child development and family studies courses. Based on Urie Bronfenbrenner's work on the ecology of human development, the book focuses on the development of competence, which Garbarino defines as the ability to succeed in life's major challenges—especially in the roles of worker, citizen, lover, and parent. Clearly written, this book is a comprehensive and thoughtful analysis of the role of the social environment in shaping children and families. As such, it is basic and important reading for all professionals who work with same.

Garbarino, James. (1995). *Raising children in a socially toxic environment.* San Francisco: Jossey-Bass.

James Garbarino created the title of his book to convey his conviction that "the mere act of living in our society today is dangerous to the health and well-being of children and adolescents." He begins by charting a dramatic decline in the quality of social life over the past 30–40 years and argues that this decline has had a profound effect on the quality of life for children and adolescents. The chapter titles read like a list of social conditions critical to healthy child development: stability, security, affirmation and acceptance, time together, values and community, and access to basic resources. Practical suggestions for parents and practitioners to counter social toxicity are included throughout. The book concludes with an A–Z list of resources and ideas for action.

Gerber, Magda, & Johnson, Allison. (1998). *Your self-confident baby: How to encourage your child's natural abilities—from the very start.* New York: Wiley.

Magda Gerber began her career in 1945 working with Dr. Emmi Pikler in Budapest, Hungary, and has been working with infants, toddlers, and their families for decades. This book is written for parents, but is also appropriate for anyone working with infants and toddlers. Magda Gerber's approach to working with infants is to get to know them as people and individuals with unique personalities and learning styles and to allow them to develop at their own pace and in their own style. In her philosophy, observing infants and toddlers before intervening will expand our capacity to respond appropriately and our children's ability to grow in competence and confidence. This "less is more" approach is a refreshing antidote to current pressures on parents to stimulate their infants from birth on in order to maximize their brain development. Although Gerber can be quite prescriptive herself at times, her basic philosophy is excellent and timeless.

Gibbs, Elizabeth, & Teti, Douglas. (Eds.). (1990). *Interdisciplinary assessment of infants: A guide for early intervention professionals.* Baltimore: Brookes.

Assessing the strengths and weaknesses of children is a challenging and uncertain science at best, and this is all the more true when assessing infants. This book takes an in-depth look at this emerging area. It begins with a section on foundations of assessment and measurement in early childhood and provides a comprehensive review of assessment of infant neuromotor integrity; cognition, language, and development; and social behavior and the social environment. Dense and scholarly in style, this book is a good resource for professionals from a variety of early intervention backgrounds who are engaged in infant assessment.

Gilkerson, Linda, Shahmoon-Shanok, Rebecca, & Pawl, Jeree. (1995). *Reflective supervision: A relationship for learning—A training videotape, discussion guide, and sourcebook.* Washington, DC: Zero to Three: National Center for Infants, Toddlers, and Families.

As its title suggests, this package includes a 60-minute videotape using role play to demonstrate the three elements central to supervision in infant/family programs—reflection, collaboration, and regularity. The accompanying discussion guide includes a transcript of the videotape, topical essays, and suggestions for using the video with various audiences. Completing the package is a Zero to Three publication, *Learning through Supervision and Mentorship: A Sourcebook* (see Fenichel above), as well as overheads for training. Supervisors will find this very helpful to their work.

Goleman, Daniel. (1995). *Emotional intelligence: Why it can matter more than IQ.* New York: Bantam Books.

Goleman, a psychologist and journalist, asserts that emotional intelligence is evidenced by qualities such as self-control, zeal and persistence, empathy, and the ability to motivate oneself. Recent studies have examined how the brain operates while we think, feel, imagine, and dream. In the first part of the book, the author describes this neurological research; Part Two describes emotional intelligence; Part Three elucidates key differences this aptitude makes; Part Four clarifies how home and school shape the emotional circuits; and Part Five documents the results of deficiencies in this realm and strategies for teaching emotional skills. This book is an excellent discussion of the roots of emotional intelligence and the particular importance of the early years in laying this foundation.

Gonzalez-Mena, Janet. (1997). *Multicultural issues in child care.* Mountain View, CA: Mayfield.

Although the title of this book implies it is written solely for child care providers, any professional working with parents or children will benefit from using this book. It focuses on how culture influences essential infant and toddler developmental issues. Chapters include communicating across cultures, toilet training, feeding and sleeping, attachment and separation, play and exploration, and socialization. Each chapter is followed by a list for further reading and detailed endnotes. It quickly becomes obvious, reading this book, that much of what appears as expert advice for parents is culture bound. Although the author does not suggest that "anything goes" in the name of cultural difference, she does stress the need for caregivers and professionals who work with parents to increase their sensitivity, communication, and problem solving around diverse child-rearing perspectives. This book provides very sound tools for doing just that.

Gonzalez-Mena, Janet, & Eyer, Dianne Widmeyer. (1997). *Infants, toddlers, and caregivers* (4th ed.). Mountain View, CA: Mayfield.

The fourth edition of this book adds information on special needs children and cross-cultural issues to its research-based focus on practical infant/toddler caregiving. Based on the "educaring" philosophy of infant specialist Magda Gerber, the book stresses the need for "three-r" interactions between caregivers and young children, that is, interactions that are respectful, responsive, and reciprocal. The book is divided into three sections by focus on the caregiver, the child, and the program, and provides comprehensive and clearly organized information throughout. Designed as a textbook for preservice training of group and family child care providers, the book is also an excellent resource for in-service training and parent education.

Gotsch, Gwen. (1994). *Breastfeeding pure and simple*. Franklin Park, IL: La Leche League International.

Published by the "grandmother" of breastfeeding information sources, La Leche League International, this book is an easy-to-read introduction to breastfeeding for new mothers or mothers who have not breastfed before. Focusing on the beginning and early months of breastfeeding and illustrated with ample photos, the book is an excellent source of basic information on this important topic. See the La Leche League International description in the Organizations/Journals section of this bibliography for ordering information.

Green, Martin I. (1994). *A sigh of relief: The first-aid handbook for childhood emergencies*. New York: Bantam Books.

This book should be an essential item in every home where young children live or visit. It begins with an excellent section on prevention, including childproofing tips; equipment safety; car, bicycle, and sports safety; and so forth. It then discusses basics of choosing a doctor and emergency room, first-aid supplies to have on hand and other basics of being prepared. The third section discusses common childhood illnesses and disorders and what to do about them. The final section addresses first-aid procedures for emergencies and accidents. The book is clearly written and attractively designed, with helpful illustrations and a comprehensive table of contents. Parents and caregivers will find this easy to read and specific, even in stressful times of emergency and illness.

Greenman, Jim. (1988). *Caring spaces, learning places: Children's environments that work*. Redmond, WA: Exchanges Press.

Designing environments for young children, particularly for infants and toddlers, is an art as well as a science. Jim Greenman has a thorough grasp of both. In addition, his obvious love for, and understanding of, infants and toddlers is apparent throughout this book. Greenman begins by making a cogent case for the fact that environments affect us pervasively and often unconsciously.

He then discusses how children learn, including a focus on the unique needs and issues of infants and toddlers in groups. Going far beyond the usual listing of equipment and floor plans often found on this topic, *Caring Spaces, Learning Places* delves into the psychology of both children and adults in group care settings and ways in which environmental design can promote positive behaviors in both. Specific chapters follow that discuss buildings and building sites; room interiors, including lighting; areas for common care routines such as eating and diapering; storage; room arrangement; and indoor and outdoor learning environments. Enhanced by attractive multicultural photographs, illustrations, and poems and quotes from both fiction and nonfiction sources, this book is a comprehensive guide to creating environments for infants, toddlers, and preschoolers that are functional, promote exploration and learning, and are fun places for adults and children to spend their time.

Greenman, Jim, & Stonehouse, Anne. (1996). *Prime times: A handbook for excellence in infant and toddler programs.* St. Paul, MN: Redleaf Press.

The authors intended this book to function as a general handbook for programs serving children under the age of 3 and as a text for students planning to work with infants and toddlers in child care. Its central philosophy is that routine caring times such as feeding, diapering, and dressing are prime times for teaching and learning. Frequently one-on-one times, these are occasions for children to learn from sensitive and responsive care that they are effective and competent human beings. Well-researched and well-organized, *Prime Times* covers almost every conceivable aspect of caregiving for infants and toddlers. Enriched throughout by the authors' obvious understanding of and love for these fascinating little people, it should be required reading for all who work with groups of infants or toddlers.

Greenspan, Stanley, & Greenspan, Nancy. (1989). *The essential partnership: How parents and children can meet the emotional challenges of infancy and childhood.* New York: Viking Penguin.

Within a framework of the six major stages of emotional growth from birth to 5 (initially described in Dr. Greenspan's earlier book, *First Feelings*), this book provides a practical guide for parents to explore their children's feelings and move toward a stronger emotional relationship. Using a variety of case examples, the book discusses how simple "floor-time" play can be used to help parents and children face challenges related to anger, sadness, fears, sexuality, competitiveness, self-esteem, and eating and sleeping patterns.

Hart, Betty, & Risley, Todd. (1995). *Meaningful differences in the everyday experience of young American children.* Baltimore: Brookes.

Summarizing 30 years of the collaborative work of two University of Kansas researchers and early interventionists, this book reads better than its topic suggests. The longitudinal study that is at the center of this book focuses on how children learn language and was based on monthly observations of 42 children and their families over a period of 2.5 years. The study began about the time the children were 1 and collected data on their language development until they were 3. The sample was evenly balanced among families using welfare supports, working-class families, and highly educated professional families. The findings show startling differences in later achievement among the children by the amount and quality of talking that went on in the household. Hart and Risley identify five categories of significant family experience that describe parenting skills of pivotal importance for children's societal competence. Both parents and early interventionists will find this book highly relevant.

Hass, Aaron. (1994). *The gift of fatherhood: How men's lives are transformed by their children.* New York: Fireside.

This book is an excellent resource for both fathers and facilitators of fathers' groups. The author is an experienced family psychologist, psychiatry professor, and father of three. Beginning with 12 common obstacles to fathering and strategies to overcome them, Hass discusses topics such as learning to love and enjoy your children more, being more patient, finding more time for children, discipline, and the marital relationship and parenting. He concludes with chapters on divorced dads and stepdads. His advice throughout is sound, practical, specific, and compelling.

Hewitt, Deborah. (1995). *So this is normal too?: Teachers and parents working out developmental issues in young children.* St. Paul, MN: Redleaf Press.

Conceived as a problem-solving approach for caregivers and parents to use together, this book is a practical resource for addressing common developmental issues. For each of 16 issues (e.g., separation, toilet training, eating habits, biting, power struggles, etc.), Hewitt defines the problem, offers suggestions for observation and problem solving, discusses how parents and providers can work together, summarizes when further help may be needed, and provides options for action.

Hewlett, Sylvia Ann, & West, Cornel. (1998). *The war against parents: What we can do for America's beleaguered moms and dads.* Boston: Houghton Mifflin.

Hewlett, a white economist, and West, a professor of religion and African American studies, have formed an effective partnership to explore what lies behind the poor life outcomes of a large proportion of American children. They argue that the parental role has been seriously eroded over the past 30 years by big business, government, and the wider culture. After making a strong case for this position over several chapters, they report on the results of a nationwide parent survey and propose specific strategies to promote a parents' bill of rights. This is a good reference for parents and all advocates for healthy families.

Honig, Alice Sterling, & Brophy, Holly Elisabeth. (1996). *Talking with your baby: Family as the first school.* Syracuse, NY: Syracuse University Press.

This book was written specifically to help low-literacy parents and those for whom English is a second language enhance the language and development of their children through daily routines at home. The 25 topical chapters are short, clearly written, and illustrated with occasional photos. *Talking with Your Baby* is a sound and easy-to-use reference for all parents of infants and the practitioners who work with them. Don't be put off by the somewhat unattractive cover and layout of the book; its content is excellent.

Hopson, Darlene Powell, & Hopson, Derek. (1990). *Different and wonderful: Raising black children in a race-conscious society.* New York: Simon & Schuster.

Authored by two black psychologists, this book was written to counter the common myth that there are no real differences between black and white children, and to emphasize the need for black parents to be positive, not simply silent, about their children's blackness. In a society where black children are still given frequent messages of inferiority, some subtle and some blatant, black parents need to counter these racist messages. The Hopsons emphasize that black children are different from white—not better, not worse, just different—and that black children can be taught to celebrate their differences. In several areas, the book calls for parents to look inward at their own feelings about race in order to be able to communicate clearly on the topic with their children. Beginning with the infant and toddler years, the authors cover common developmental issues and their racial overtones and implications for black families throughout the child-rearing years. The book is pleasant reading and loaded with sound and practical information.

Huggins, Kathleen. (1995). *The nursing mother's companion.* Boston: Harvard Common Press.

Breastfeeding is widely recognized as the most healthy and natural way to feed an infant. Yet it is not commonly practiced by mothers, and its techniques are not commonly understood by pediatricians. In this book, Kathleen Huggins, a registered nurse and lactation consultant, provides a thorough explanation of effective breastfeeding techniques from the first week, through the first 2 months, from 2 to 6 months, and for nursing the older baby and toddler. In each section, she discusses common problems and how to overcome them. Nursing while working outside the home is discussed, as is nursing twins and infants with special needs. Supplemented by beautiful photographs by Harriette Hartigan and clear illustrations, this book is an excellent resource for nursing mothers and professionals who work with them.

Ilse, Sherokee. (1990). *Empty arms: Coping with miscarriage, stillbirth and infant death*. Maple Plain, MN: Wintergreen Press.

As its title indicates, this book was written as a resource for parents who have experienced the death of an unborn, newborn, or infant child. Written by a woman who delivered a full-term stillborn child and experienced two miscarriages, as well as birthing two living sons, this book is an empathic and solid resource for grieving parents. It begins by discussing the first stage of learning about a baby's death through a variety of different circumstances. It reviews decisions parents will face immediately, such as whether to view and hold their child, considering an autopsy, and funeral arrangements. It examines issues at different stages of grieving, and what family and friends can do. It concludes with an extensive annotated resource list of organizations, publications, and audiovisual materials addressing the grief of coping with infant loss.

Johnson, Anne, & Goodman, Vic. (1995). *The essence of parenting*. New York: Crossroad.

Consisting of 23 short chapters, this book is designed to be read and reread slowly and thoughtfully. Although brief, each chapter is also quite pithy, and the authors encourage readers to pause and reflect as they go along. The book focuses on our state of mind as we interact with, discipline, and nurture our children. What we model to our children speaks much louder than any words or techniques we use. If we want our children to recognize and handle their feelings in healthy ways, to be empathetic and treat others with respect, and to realize their potential for learning and growing, it all begins with how we nourish and model these qualities in ourselves. The authors make a compelling case that who we *are*, not what we *do*, is the essence of parenting. Excellent for parents and anyone who works with parents, this book is wise and profound in its simplicity.

Kagan, Sharon L. (1991). *United we stand: Collaboration for child care and early education services*. New York: Teachers College Press.

This concise and well-written book defines collaboration and discusses its historical context, its rationale and benefits, and stages in its process. An underlying premise is that collaboration is not a panacea to systemic problems in early care and education, but a means to the end of minimizing weaknesses while maximizing system effectiveness. Kagan reviews challenges and limitations and examines elements of successful collaborations. The book concludes with a descriptive listing of existing collaborations with contact information.

Kennedy, Marge, & King, Janet Spencer. (1994). *The single-parent family: Living happily in a changing world*. New York: Crown Trade Paperbacks.

The authors state that according to the 1990 census, close to one in three households in the United States is headed by a single parent. Yet many parent education books and programs seem to assume the presence of two parents.

Written by two single parents who interviewed and surveyed hundreds of others, with each chapter including a section called the "professional point of view," this book is a practical and comprehensive resource for single parents and the professionals who work with them. It covers topics such as taking care of yourself, establishing the foundation for family life, family management methods, and household management basics. It also includes a discussion of new and old family rituals, and suggestions to single parents for creating a life of their own. *The Single-Parent Family* is well organized and inclusive of many important specifics.

Kitzinger, Sheila. (1989). *The crying baby*. London: Penguin Books.

Sheila Kitzinger has studied and written prolifically on the topics of pregnancy, childbirth, mothering, and female sexuality in many cultures. In her foreword, she asserts that there is a great deal of female knowledge about babies in the Third World, traditional cultures, and the industrial West that is not contained in the many parenting books written by experts. She wrote this book after surveying 1,400 women in Australia and Britain. The book begins by describing the impact of a crying baby and giving an overview of the reasons babies cry. Separate chapters then discuss a variety of causes for a baby's crying and offer a variety of mother-tested strategies for dealing with them. The last chapter of the book describes parent–child practices in other cultures. One of the most striking differences between many so-called Third World and traditional societies and our modern Western culture is the manner in which mothers and their newborns are treated. As Kitzinger describes it, in traditional societies, mothers of newborns are cherished and nurtured by female relatives and friends for up to 6 weeks or more. These mothers in a sense get their batteries charged, the better to nurture and cherish their babies. The isolation of mothers in our Western culture contributes to the agony and frustration of dealing with a constantly crying baby; the tenseness of the mother aggravates the baby's discomfort, and a vicious cycle ensues. *The Crying Baby* offers practical strategies and a wealth of reassurance that can help to head off or break this negative cycle.

Klass, Carol S. (1996). *Home visiting: Promoting healthy parent and child development*. Baltimore: Brookes.

This handbook is a terrific addition to the limited volume of literature written specifically for home visitors. The author has had over 20 years of experience and research in helping parents and teachers of young children improve their caregiving skills. She identifies three themes central to home visiting, which frame the book's content: (1) development occurs within and through relationship, (2) all relationship involves mutuality, and (3) child and parent development are intertwined with their social environment. The first third of the book focuses on the relationship between parents and the home visitor, skills required for home visiting, and training and supervision issues. The remainder of the book is devoted to a clearly presented and well-researched discussion of developmental issues pertinent to parents of young children. Enlivened throughout by vignettes of skilled home visitors in action and concluding with an appendix of resources for home visitors, *Home Visiting* is a must-have reference for home visitors from all disciplines who work with families of children aged birth to 5.

Klaus, Marshall, & Klaus, Phyllis. (1998). *Your amazing newborn.* Reading, MA: Perseus Books.

Health care professionals, home visitors, and other practitioners who work with families of newborns will find this book an invaluable addition to their libraries. Written for parents, the detailed text is clear and engaging. The heart of the book, however, is the collection of stunning black-and-white photos of ethnically diverse newborns with their parents and grandparents, which complement the text beautifully. Chapter topics include the minutes and hours after childbirth, and the newborn capacities for sight, hearing, touch, taste, smell, movement, emotional expression, and imitation. Helpful chapters on the newly adopted baby and the newborn family conclude the book.

Koch, Tina, & Kamberg, Mary-Lane. (1995). *Tips from Tina: Help around the house—Hundreds of practical ideas to make family child care easier and more fun.* St. Paul, MN: Redleaf Press.

The title of this book clearly describes what it is, and it is very practical indeed. With chapters on kitchen, dining room, pantry, living room, bedroom, bathroom, closets, office, playroom/basement, garage, and yard, every area of a family child care provider's home is addressed. Tina Koch is an experienced family child care provider, and her experience shows. The layout of the book lends itself to quick and easy reading, a plus for busy child care providers.

Koch, Tina, & Kamberg, Mary-Lane. (1997). *Cabin fever relievers: Hundreds of games, activities, and crafts for creative indoor fun.* St. Paul, MN: Redleaf Press.

Another excellent resource for family child care providers or for parents, this book is particularly helpful for cold or rainy climates. It can be a sanity saver with a group of wiggly toddlers on a frigid winter or scorching summer day. The activities include creative approaches to arts and crafts, movement, music, water play, active movement games, and more.

Kotulak, Ronald. (1996). *Inside the brain: Revolutionary discoveries of how the mind works.* Kansas City, MO: Andrews and McMeel.

There is a flurry of interest in the current research on brain development and its implications for the first 3 years of life. This Pulitzer Prize-winning science writer has synthesized interviews with more than 300 neuroscientists into a book dedicated to all parents and teachers. The book is divided into three sections: "How the brain gets built," "How the brain gets damaged," and "How the brain fixes itself." Kotulak writes clearly and uses frequent metaphors (e.g., "Long thought to be a clean slate . . . the brain is now seen as a super-sponge that is most absorbent from birth to about the age of twelve") to translate scientific data into a form comprehensible to the layperson. This is a very helpful summary of research pivotal to the early childhood field.

Kunhardt, Jean, Spiegel, Lisa, & Basile, Sandra. (1996). *Mother's circle: Wisdom and reassurance from other mothers on your first year with baby.* New York: Avon Books.

Written by two experienced parent group leaders and a parent writer, this book distills the experiences of a group of New York City mothers during the first year of their babies lives. The chapter topics focus on issues common to this period and include loving your baby and the fear of spoiling, work and motherhood, feeding and nurturing, changes in your marriage, changes in your body, babies and sleep, your mother's legacy, and attachment and separation. These mothers all appear to be upper-middle-class, educated, married women. Parents from similar socioeconomic backgrounds are likely to find this book reassuring and helpful. The chapter on sleep comes across as very opinionated, but other chapters are balanced. This book would also be a good resource for parent educators working with mother–infant groups.

Lally, J. Ron, Griffin, Abbey, Fenichel, Emily, Segal, Marilyn, Szanton, Eleanor Stokes, & Weissbourd, Bernice. (1995). *Caring for infants and toddlers in groups: Developmentally appropriate practice.* Washington, DC: Zero to Three.

This clear and practical guide is designed to help practitioners offer a nurturing group care environment for very young children. Beginning with an overview of typical infant and toddler development, it features examples of appropriate and inappropriate caregiver responses to a wide range of issues and situations typically encountered in group care of infants and toddlers. The guide is illustrated with many attractive photos and offers a concise chart of developmental milestones for children from birth to age 3. Concluding with references and resources for further reading, *Caring for Infants and Toddlers in Groups* is essential reading for anyone involved in same.

Lappe, Frances Moore, & Dubois, Paul Martin. (1994). *The quickening of America: Rebuilding our nation, remaking our lives.* San Francisco: Jossey-Bass.

This book focuses on community efforts across the nation that are developing solutions from within to problems in local schools, workplaces, and neighborhoods. One of its major premises is that social and personal change are intertwined, and that each of us as an individual is capable of making a difference—a refreshing antidote to the widespread cynicism and hopelessness that seems to characterize the current mood of our nation's citizenry. Several promising initiatives are profiled in the book, and practical tools for energizing ourselves and our communities are discussed. *The Quickening of America* offers both parents and interventionists idealistic yet pragmatic alternatives to discouragement and apathy.

Leach, Penelope. (1994). *Children first: What our society must do—and is not doing—for our children today.* New York: Knopf.

In this book, the British author of the classic *Your Baby and Child* argues compellingly that our Western society is unfriendly, even inimical, to the development of children and families. She begins with an economic perspective and then moves through the developmental stages of children's lives, illuminating the conflicts between children's needs and societal pressures. The final section of the book proposes new approaches to poverty and privilege, human rights for children, working and caring, and practical parenting. This book is dense reading, but very thought provoking. It gives a whole new meaning to the words "family values." Although this book may appear to be a radical departure from Dr. Leach's previous baby and child care books, its themes and underlying passion are consistent with her earlier work. Throughout, she is a sensitive observer of and respondent to the cues of the baby and child, has a broad and inclusive cultural perspective, and offers readers the tools to become more sensitive, aware, and effective parents. In addition, *Children First* offers parents and professionals tools for becoming more effective child advocates in the larger society.

Leach, Penelope. (1997). *Your baby and child: From birth to age five.* New York: Knopf.

If there is one book that embodies sound child-rearing advice, while being practical, comprehensive, and beautiful, this is it. *Your Baby and Child* is a terrific resource for both new and experienced parents. The latest revision, like earlier versions, is clearly organized, with bountiful, full-color, multicultural photographs throughout. Beginning with the birth process, most of the book is devoted to care of the newborn, growing infant, and toddler, with the final section of the book focused on the preschool child. Throughout, the author sensitizes the reader to the child's perspective on normal developmental issues and everyday care. If parents and parent educators could own only one book on early childhood development, this would be the one to buy.

Leffert, Nancy, Benson, Peter, & Roehlkepartain, Jolene. (1997). *Starting out right: Developmental assets for children.* Minneapolis: Search Institute.

In 1990, Search Institute introduced the concept of developmental assets for adolescents based on a survey study of 47,000 6th- to 12th-grade students across the United States. Since then, the Institute's research has documented that the more of these assets young people have, the less likely they are to engage in negative behaviors. In this report, the Institute traces the roots of the 40 assets it identified and adapts the framework for infants and toddlers, preschoolers, and elementary-age children. The adaptation process blended an extensive review of literature with input from practitioners and experts in the early childhood field. A fresh and clearly written summary, this report is a good resource for the "strengths-based" approach to serving families.

LeShan, Eda. (1993). *Grandparenting in a changing world.* New York: New-market Press.

Eda LeShan writes this book in the first person with an easy-to-read, conversational style. She recognizes that children today are growing up in a vastly different world than many of their parents and that the role of grandparents must change to address these changes. Her book is comprehensive and covers basic grandparenting issues as well as situations of divorce, crisis, and grandparents raising their grandchildren. Her theme throughout is that the central role of grandparents is to provide unconditional love, as well as to model for their grandchildren what it means to be an ethical, moral, caring person. Concluding with a resource list and helpful bibliography, this book is an eloquent, contemporary portrayal of the crucial role grandparents can play in the lives of their grandchildren.

Levine, James A., Murphy, Dennis T., & Wilson, Sherrill. (1993). *Getting men involved: Strategies for early childhood programs.* New York: Scholastic.

As its title indicates, this book is a compendium of strategies for involving fathers and other significant males in early childhood programming. Less research-based than the Minnesota Fathering Alliance book also listed in this bibliography, it is more of a smorgasbord of ideas from successful programs around the country. *Getting Men Involved* includes a "Male Involvement Profile" that provides thoughtful questions through which programs can assess their efforts (or lack of same) to reach beyond involving only women in their activities. Although some may find the format a bit busy and the organization a bit fuzzy, the book has many good ideas for involving fathers and other significant men in the lives of their children. It concludes with an extensive resource section on books for children and printed materials that will be helpful to professionals and parents.

Levine, James, & Pitt, Edward W. (1995). *New expectations: Community strategies for responsible fatherhood.* New York: Families and Work Institute.

The increasing numbers of single-parent families headed by women and the simultaneous trend of fathers becoming more involved in child caring are drawing wide public attention to the role of fathers in children's lives. This comprehensive publication includes a review of father-related research, descriptions of current community-based strategies, tips from leading practitioners, a guide to fathering programs nationwide, an annotated bibliography of current publications in the field, and great photographs of fathers and children. A central theme of the book is that high expectations and attitudinal change on the part of agencies and society in general will go a long way toward increasing the involvement of fathers in children's lives.

Lieberman, Alicia. (1993). *The emotional life of the toddler.* New York: Free Press.

Building on the author's experience as an attachment researcher and parent–infant psychotherapist, this book is a thoughtful look at the emotional life of children from 1 to 3 years of age. It covers such issues as the challenges of being and living with a toddler, temperamental differences, active toddlers, shy toddlers, early anxieties, common developmental concerns, toddlers and divorce, and toddlers in child care. Enriched by vignettes and case studies, this book provides parents and practitioners with a comprehensive window into the emotions of these intriguing small people.

Lindsay, Jeanne Warren. (1993). *Teen dads: Rights, responsibilities, and joys.* Buena Park, CA: Morning Glory Press.

One of an extensive series of well-written books for teen parents by this author and publisher, *Teen Dads* is illustrated throughout with beautiful multiethnic photos of actual teen parents and their babies. It focuses on the basics of parenting, beginning with pregnancy and continuing through the first 3 years. Quotes from teen fathers enrich the text, which is sound, comprehensive, and attractively simple. This book will be very helpful for teen fathers and mothers and the people who work with them.

Littell, Julia H. (1986). *Building strong foundations: Evaluation strategies for family resource programs.* Chicago: Family Resource Coalition.

This book, much more basic than the Weiss and Jacobs book discussed elsewhere in this list, is an excellent resource for beginners in program evaluation. It begins by addressing the need and uses for evaluation, then clearly discusses basic concepts and steps in the evaluation process. It clarifies the difference between formative and summative evaluation and reviews strategies for each. A glossary of terms, list of suggested readings, and sample data collection forms conclude the book. This book is one of several excellent publications available from the Family Resource Coalition of America, a national organization whose goal is to improve the content and expand the number of programs available to parents across the country.

Lynch, Eleanor, & Hanson, Marci. (Eds.). (1998). *Developing cross-cultural competence: A guide for working with children and their families.* Baltimore: Brookes.

Edited by two special education professors, this book was written to enhance the delivery of early intervention services to families from a wide variety

of cultural and ethnic backgrounds. It will be helpful to service providers from
health, education, and social services. Beginning with persuasive information on
the need for interventionists to become culturally competent, the book continues
with basic strategies for doing so, followed by chapters written from a broad
variety of cultural perspectives. These focus on families with European, Native
American, African, Latino, Asian, Filipino, Native Hawaiian and Pacific Island,
and Middle Eastern roots. Each of the culturally specific chapters concludes with
appendices summarizing contrasting beliefs, values, and practices; cultural cour-
tesies and customs; significant cultural holidays, events, and practices; and some
basic vocabulary concepts. A helpful suggested reading list of fiction and nonfiction with cultural themes concludes the book.

Martin, Elaine. (1988). *Baby games: The joyful guide to child's play from birth
to three years.* Philadelphia: Running Press.

Designed for parents, this is a lovely collection of play activities for infants,
toddlers, and preschoolers, all in one book. Organized by 3-month age spreads
up to 18 months and 6-month spans from 18 to 36 months, the chapters each
begin with an overview of typical developmental steps and issues for that age
group. Then a wide variety of activities are suggested for routine daily events,
such as dressing and eating. Indoor and outdoor activities, music, art, and movement are included for each age level. The book concludes with suggestions for
books, musical recordings, toys, and party ideas.

McClure, Vimala Schneider. (1989). *Infant massage: A handbook for loving parents.* New York: Bantam Books.

The importance of loving touch to the healthy development of young children has been proven by research. In today's climate of high stress and achievement orientation, the importance of this basic factor may be even more important and less self-evident. Vimala McClure begins by reviewing the worldwide
commonality of infant massage and discusses how it contributes to the critical
attachment process between parent and child. She discusses how to set the stage
for massage and then goes through step-by-step strategies for full body massage
of infants. Included are variations for illness and colic, premature babies, special
needs babies, and older children. Augmented by words and music to multicultural lullabies, rhymes and games for older babies, and multiple photographs,
this book is a comprehensive and clearly written handbook for parents and service providers who are interested in expanding their repertoire of effective adult–
child communication techniques.

McGoldrick, Monica, Giordano, Joe, & Pearce, John K. (Eds.). (1996). *Ethnicity and family therapy* (2nd ed.). New York: Guilford Press.

Written for mental health professionals, the first edition of this book was
one of the early resources for cultural competency and served as a comprehensive and helpful resource for professionals in other human service fields as well.

It discusses the progression in family therapy from focus on the individual to focus on the family to focus on the larger environment of culture. An analogy is that therapists are using an expanding wide-angle lens with which to view families. One of the interesting features of this book is its examination of various cultures within the Anglo-European umbrella, a reminder of the infinite diversity of culture, even within broad ethnic groups. Completely revised and expanded, the second edition begins with a broad conceptual overview and describes cultural variations of over 40 different ethnic groups in separate chapters. Throughout, the book maintains a respectful tone while examining variations in family values and gender issues across cultures. It also cautions against overgeneralizing cultural commonalities or differences and overlooking individual differences. In today's rapidly changing world, *Ethnicity and Family Therapy* has become an essential resource for all practitioners working with families.

Meisels, Samuel J., & Fenichel, Emily. (Eds.). (1996). *New visions for the developmental assessment of infants and young children.* Washington, DC: Zero to Three.

Clearly written and comprehensive in scope, this book offers a state-of-the-art review of assessment theory and practice designed to strengthen understanding of very young children's skills and abilities in order to help them reach their developmental potential. It includes principles and guidelines for developmental assessment, how to incorporate the perspectives of parents, guidelines on the importance of sociocultural background, new approaches to assessment, and the impact of public policies on assessment and intervention.

Meisels, Samuel J., & Shonkoff, Jack P. (Eds.). (1990). *Handbook of early childhood intervention.* New York: Cambridge University Press.

The most comprehensive reference on the topic of early intervention currently available in a single volume, this handbook is an excellent addition to the bookshelf of all professionals who work in the field of early childhood intervention. An edited collection of the work of persons such as James Garbarino, Carl Dunst, Kathryn Barnard, Linda Gilkerson, Robert Halpern, Peggy Pizzo, and others, the *Handbook* represents the best thinking of many of the leaders in the field. The book begins with a historical overview on early intervention, and section titles include Concepts of Developmental Vulnerability, Theoretical Bases of Early Intervention, Approaches to Assessment, Models of Service Delivery, Research Perspectives and Findings, and Policy Issues and Programmatic Directions. Extensive reference lists follow each chapter, and comprehensive name and subject indexes conclude the volume.

Melina, Lois Ruskai. (1986). *Raising adoptive children: A manual for adoptive parents.* New York: Harper Perennial.

Lois Melina is an adoptive parent, journalist, lecturer, and editor of a national adoption newsletter. She is also skilled at making research findings and their implications for caregiving intelligible to lay people. Although only the first section of the book specifically addresses infant and toddler issues, the book contains a wealth of information that is essential for all parents of adopted children. These include topics such as the family medical history, talking with children about adoption, adoption's effects on the family, transracial family issues, and dealing with serious behavior problems and special adoption situations. Solid information is provided on dealing with children with attachment disorders. *Raising Adoptive Children* is an excellent resource for adoptive parents and the professionals who work with them.

Miller, Nancy B. (1994). *Nobody's perfect: Living and growing with children who have special needs.* Baltimore: Brookes.

Written by a support group facilitator for parents of children with special needs, this is a rich, fresh, and very grounded resource for parents. Four stages of adaptation to having a child with special needs are identified: surviving, searching, settling in, and separating. Strategies for successful adaptation in all four stages are described comprehensively and empathetically. The author has 25 years of experience counseling families with children who have special needs, and this experience shows.

Minnesota Extension Service & University of Wisconsin Extension. (1995). *Positive parenting.* Minneapolis: University of Minnesota.

This video-based parent education curriculum focuses on alternatives to physical punishment in the discipline of children. Developed jointly by family educators at two major universities, the curriculum includes six lesson units, each consisting of a video (about 10 minutes), parent handouts, a teacher/leader guide, discussion aids, and a related reference list. Specific topics include nonviolent discipline strategies, the importance of both love and limits, natural and logical consequences, reflective listening, how to deal with your own and your child's anger, and tactics for dealing with oppositional behavior. Although the curriculum addresses parenting issues that extend well into the elementary school years, the information on the infant and toddler period is useful. And the overall philosophy of peaceful parenting will be helpful to new parents as they develop effective ways to guide and encourage their growing child.

The Minnesota Fathering Alliance. (1992). *Working with fathers.* Stillwater, MN: nu ink unlimited.

Designed for professionals who work with parents, this book clearly recognizes that working with fathers in parent education settings is different from working with mothers. It begins with a comprehensive literature review on men and fatherhood, discusses cultural influences on fathers, and examines the basics of working with fathers, such as planning programs and father–child activity times, group leadership issues, issues to address when women facilitate all-male groups, and parent education methods that are effective with men. It then has separate chapters on working with single fathers; gay fathers; young, unmarried fathers; and fathers with special needs children. *Working with Fathers* was written by a team of 16 persons experienced in working with male parents and coedited by two long-time parent educators in Minnesota's Early Childhood Family Education programs. It is a well-organized, clearly written, excellent resource for anyone working with fathers.

Morris, Linda Rappaport, & Schulz, Linda. (1989). *Creative play activities for children with disabilities: A resource book for teachers and parents.* Champaign, IL: Human Kinetics Books.

Beginning with a chapter of very helpful tips for successful playtimes and suggested considerations for children who are deaf or hearing impaired, blind or visually impaired, or physically impaired, this book is an encyclopedia of play ideas. Chapters on sensory games, movement, water play, outdoors, make-believe, arts and crafts, music and rhythm, and group activities include clear directions and required "ingredients." This collection is equally useful for parents and interventionists.

Naseef, Robert. (1997). *Special children, challenged parents: The struggles and rewards of raising a child with a disability.* Secaucus, NJ: Carol.

As a parent of a child with autism and a psychologist whose specialty is counseling families of special needs children, this author is well grounded in his subject. He suggests that the central issue for these parents is coping with the fact that their children will not lead the life the parents wanted for them. Naseef covers a wide range of topics including dealing with the first impact of having a child with a disability, working through grief, tuning in day by day to your child, guiding behavior, fathers and grief, couples' issues, siblings' issues, building support circles, and dealing with professionals and interventionists. He also provides a list of telephone and online resources and an helpful bibliography for parents and practitioners. Laced with anecdotes from personal experience (his own and that of his clients), this book is eloquent and insightful. It is an outstanding resource for parents, but would also be very useful for parent educators and interventionists.

Nelsen, Jane, Erwin, Cheryl, & Delzer, Carol. (1994). *Positive discipline for single parents: A practical guide to raising children who are responsible, respectful, and resourceful.* Rocklin, CA: Prima.

Recognizing that most of the books on discipline assume the presence of two parents raising children together, this book focuses on the special issues of single parents in relation to discipline. Two of the three authors are single parents, and their experience shows. Although not as comprehensive or specific as Sears and Sears' *The Discipline Book*, the central thesis is the same: that effective discipline is based on a foundation of love and healthy relationship. The authors discuss positive discipline strategies within the overall perspective that single parenting has unique strengths and assets. Whether living with a partner or single, parents who are willing to learn, are not afraid to make mistakes, and try their best without expecting perfection can raise healthy, well-adjusted children.

Newman, Margaret. (1994). *Stepfamily realities*. Oakland, CA: New Harbinger.

Stepfamilies are much more complex entities than nonblended families. Children are on the scene from the beginning. Partners bring more separate history and do not have the opportunity to create their family without children. Written by a psychologist and marriage counselor who is a stepparent herself, this book addresses common issues that arise in stepfamilies such as discipline, boundaries, sexuality, rituals and habits, jealousy, sibling displacement, money issues, changed relationships, and biological children. Concluding with two chapters on assertive communication, this book is a very helpful guide to parents and interventionists immersed in the issues of stepfamilies.

Nugent, J. Kevin. (1985). *Using the NBAS with infants and their families*. White Plains, NY: March of Dimes Birth Defects Foundation. (out of print)

The Neonatal Behavioral Assessment Scale (NBAS) was developed by T. Berry Brazelton and colleagues at Boston Children's Hospital Medical Center and published in 1973. According to Dr. Brazelton, its original purpose was to assist professionals in promoting parent–infant attachment. The NBAS offers a comprehensive picture of babies and their behavior. When a trained examiner works with newborns in the presence of their parents, parents can gain insights into how their baby deals with the world. Although this book is designed for use by trained clinicians, it is also useful for other professionals and parents to gain insights into the remarkable capacities of a newborn. For each of the 27 items on the NBAS (e.g., rooting and sucking, other infant reflexes, cuddliness, irritability and consolability), the book describes the item and the infant's response, interprets the developmental significance of the behavior, describes the developmental sequence of the behavior through the first months of life, and offers possible implications for caregiving.

Pantell, Robert, Fries, James, & Vickery, Donald. (1998). *Taking care of your child: A parent's guide to complete medical care*. Reading, MA: Addison-Wesley.

Winner of the American Medical Writers Association Book Award and revised and updated regularly, this book is an excellent overall health reference for parents of children prenatally through adolescence. About half the book consists of informative text on child development and common health issues. The remainder consists of decision charts for common medical emergencies, injuries, and illnesses. The charts are clearly written and spell out common symptoms, when and how to use home treatment, and when and how fast to contact a doctor. Each chart concludes with a discussion of what to expect at the doctor's office. A comprehensive index makes locating information a fast and easy process.

Parks, Stephanie, Furuno, Setsu, O'Reilly, Katherine, Inatsuka, Takayo, Hosaka, Carol, & Zeisloft-Falbey, Barbara. (1998). *HELP at home (birth–3)*. Palo Alto, CA: VORT Corporation.

Based on the Hawaii Early Learning Profile (HELP), this three-ring binder version is an updated and adapted version of the original *HELP Activity Guide*. Newly formatted, these developmental activity sheets for each of the 685 developmental skills identified in the HELP checklist are designed for professionals to copy and give to parents of children developing in the birth–36-month age range. Each activity sheet begins with an introduction to the developmental skill being addressed and is written from the baby's or child's point of view. Activities follow for parents to initiate with their child to promote the development of that specific skill, and the sheets conclude with a space for notes. Each activity sheet is contained on one page and includes a photograph or illustration. The activity sheets are chronologically arranged by age in six categories—cognitive, language, gross motor, fine motor, social, and self-help—and often cross-reference activity sheets in other categories. Designed for any professional working with parents and young children, *HELP at Home* is a comprehensive, practical, and useful resource.

Pinderhughes, Elaine. (1989). *Understanding race, ethnicity, and power: The key to efficacy in clinical practice*. New York: Free Press.

Written by a social work professor and experienced cultural sensitivity trainer, this book far surpasses the typical survey approach to cultural competence. It concentrates internally on the practitioner's own life experience and cultural heritage. Separate and thought-provoking chapters focus on understanding the concepts of difference, ethnicity, race, and power. Using concrete examples throughout, the author then applies this knowledge of cultural dynamics to working with diverse clientele. This book should be required reading for all health, education, and human service professionals.

Pipher, Mary. (1996). *The shelter of each other: Rebuilding our families*. New York: Ballantine Books.

Mary Pipher is a Midwestern psychologist in private practice and is on the national lecture circuit since publication of her book *Reviving Ophelia*. In this book, she focuses on contemporary pressures that work against healthy, well-functioning families. She begins by describing how intense workplace pressures, the omnipresent television, video games, consumerism, and so forth impair family functioning and illustrates her points with anecdotes from her therapeutic practice. Pipher also targets misguided therapeutic approaches that focus on internal family dysfunction as the root of all problems. She then describes attributes of well-functioning families and how therapists and interventionists can support and promote these attributes. The book concludes with strategies families can use to protect themselves while building supportive communities in which to thrive.

Ramey, Craig, & Ramey, Sharon. (1999). *Right from birth: Building your child's foundation for life, birth to 18 months.* New York: Goddard Press.

This book is coauthored by a husband-and-wife professional team who write from their combined perspective as parents and grandparents and as researchers who have worked with thousands of young children and families over three decades. In the first section of the book, *Right from Birth* reviews the findings of recent brain research and how science is changing the way we parent. This discussion is followed by overviews of the latest research on how infants learn, the foundation of trust, social and emotional development, language and communication, intelligence, behavior guidance, and good child care. All of these topics are accurately, completely, and clearly covered in understandable language. The second section of the book applies this knowledge in six well-organized, age-related chapters from birth to 18 months. An excellent and timely addition to the literature for parents and practitioners, this book is flawed only by the fact that its attractive photos are not very ethnically diverse.

Rosenblith, Judy F. (1995). *In the beginning: Development from conception to age two.* Newbury Park, CA: Sage.

Although this book was designed as a textbook for undergraduate and graduate students in a variety of fields and is an expensive hardcover book, it is an excellent resource for professionals working with infants and their parents. Beginning with a historical introduction to the study of infants, the book proceeds methodically through the conception through birth period and the effects of genetic and environmental factors on infant constitution and parent–infant interaction. It continues with detailed discussion of the early characteristics and development of infants; the processes of cognitive, language, and social development; and the influence of environment on development and parent–child interaction during the first 2 years of life. Throughout, *In the Beginning* synthesizes historical and research perspectives in a clearly written style. In short, this book provides more than most infant practitioners would ever need to know about infants, with astoundingly extensive reference lists provided after each chapter.

Rothenberg, B. Annye, Hitchcock, Sandra, Harrison, Mary Lou, & Graham, Melinda. (1995). *Parentmaking: A practical handbook for teaching parent classes about babies and toddlers.* Menlo Park, CA: Banster Press.

There are not many resources for parent educators that combine the theory and practice of adult education with specific theory and practice of caring for infants and toddlers in a readily usable format. Loaded with practical information, teaching methods, and reproducible handouts and worksheets, this book is a terrific resource for anyone teaching infant and toddler parenting classes. Like any comprehensive curriculum, this is best used as a resource, not as a rote recipe for parent classes. The *Parentmaking* handbook is a very affordable and helpful resource. (Additionally, Rothenberg et al. have produced a video-based training program for early childhood parent educators. Although the information presented is sound, the videos appear amateurish and are difficult to watch. The training program must be purchased as a package and is quite expensive.)

Samalin, Nancy, with Whitney, Catherine. (1991). *Love and anger: The parental dilemma*. New York: Penguin Books.

As parents, we are sometimes shocked and appalled at the rage our children can evoke in us. Adding the findings of a parent survey on anger to her experience as a long-time facilitator of parent workshops, Nancy Samalin addresses the phenomena of parental love and anger with specificity and skill. With multiple anecdotes, she addresses dealing with anger when our children do not cooperate with reasonable routines, when they defy us, when siblings fight, when we are parenting without a partner, and when our children disappoint us. She discusses rage that edges into abuse and how to accept and handle our angry feelings. The book concludes with eight helpful tools for managing confrontations with our children.

Sammons, William A., & Lewis, Jennifer M. (1985). *Premature babies: A different beginning*. St. Louis, MO: Mosby.

Written by two pediatricians with many years of experience in intensive care nurseries, this book is a comprehensive resource for parents and professionals working with premature babies and their families. After a brief history of premature infant care, the book begins with a discussion of the pregnancy period and its function as a time of preparation and planning for the baby to come. It stresses that the final 4–6 weeks of pregnancy are a vital phase of practical, physiological, and emotional preparation for the baby. Thus the premature birth of a baby often results in the premature parent(s) feeling unprepared and shaky. Ensuing chapters cover a broad range of topics such as the neonatal intensive care unit (NICU), development of the premature infant, discharge from the NICU, the parents' and the infant's perspective on going home, sleep, feeding, siblings, twins, support groups, and medical problems and procedures. Throughout, *Premature Babies* stresses that these babies not only have an earlier beginning, but a *different* beginning. Its clear discussion of these differences and their implications for care should be reassuring to parents and the professionals with whom they interact.

Satter, Ellyn. (1987). *How to get your kid to eat . . . But not too much*. Palo Alto, CA: Bull.

Written by a therapist specializing in the treatment of eating disorders, who has also authored *Child of Mine: Feeding with Love and Good Sense*, this book is a comprehensive resource that focuses on how to get children to develop healthy eating habits. Satter begins by clarifying her basic principles on feeding. Parents are responsible for what food is presented and the manner in which it is presented. Children are responsible for how much and even whether they eat. She discusses why pressure tactics don't work and can lead to unhealthy attitudes about food. The importance of healthy snacks is addressed. Subsequent chapters deal with specifics of feeding newborns, older babies, toddlers, preschoolers, school-age children, and teenagers. The book concludes with chapters on special feeding problems. Although this author's writing style could be better edited, the content is sound and helpful.

Schorr, Lisbeth. (1997). *Common purpose: Strengthening families and neighborhoods to rebuild America.* New York: Anchor Books.

Schorr, the author of *Within Our Reach,* outdoes her earlier work in this extensive, specific, and optimistic review of how community members, policymakers, the private sector, and others can unite to improve the lives of families and children. She begins by examining the research on successful programs and discusses ideas and experiments for reforming welfare, child protection, and public education. *Common Purpose* concludes with how all this knowledge can inform efforts to transform and rebuild neighborhoods and communities to provide better support for children and families.

Sears, William. (1985). *Nighttime parenting: How to get your baby and child to sleep.* New York: New American Library.

Dr. William Sears, a pediatrician and father of a large family, consistently promotes the practice of what he terms "attachment parenting." One of the practices of attachment parenting that he describes at length in this book is parents sharing sleep with their babies. Worldwide, it is more common for parents to sleep with their children than separately from them. Sears argues that many of what we consider sleep problems and disturbances are actually normal sleep patterns for babies and young children, and that the common practice of separating babies for night sleeping is what turns these normal patterns into problems. He offers specific suggestions for getting babies to sleep and dealing with night waking that are practical and easy to implement and that recognize the universal infant need for close bodily contact with adults. The techniques described in *Nighttime Parenting* are offered as alternatives, not as the one, right way to parent, and are a helpful addition to the literature on this topic.

Sears, William, & Sears, Martha. (1993). *The baby book: Everything you need to know about your baby from birth to age two.* Boston: Little, Brown.

The Baby Book is authored by William and Martha Sears, two pediatric specialists and parents of a large family. It focuses on five general baby care areas: eating, sleeping, development, health, and comfort, with comprehensive information offered in all areas. Sections on self-help home health care, lifesaving, and first aid for emergencies are also included. Attractive illustrations add to the text, but could be more culturally diverse. If a parent could afford only one baby care book, this might be the best choice, with its thorough and current information clearly presented.

Sears, William, & Sears, Martha. (1995). *The discipline book: Everything you need to know to have a better-behaved child—from birth to age ten.* Boston: Little, Brown.

Once again, William and Martha Sears have written an excellent, comprehensive, and well-grounded resource for parents—in this case, addressing the thorny topic of discipline. They promote what they call the attachment approach to discipline, which they say includes the good features of other styles, such as the authoritarian style, the communication approach, and the behavior modification approach. It also judiciously includes punishment and consequences. They base the discussion throughout the book on ten basic principles: get connected early, know your child, help your child to respect authority, set limits and provide structure, expect obedience, model discipline, nurture your child's self-confidence, shape your child's behavior, raise kids who care, and talk and listen.

Seligman, Milton, & Darling, Rosalyn Benjamin. (1997). *Ordinary families, special children: A systems approach to childhood disability* (2nd ed.). New York: Guilford Press.

Written for professionals in education, social work, pediatrics, and other human service areas, this book is an excellent resource for effectively working with children with disabilities in the context of their families and larger social environments. It begins with a conceptual framework on family systems theory and systematically addresses the first and continuing reactions of parents when they have a disabled child. It examines the effects on the family as a system, on siblings, and on fathers and grandparents. The focus then shifts to systemic models of intervention, cultural variations, working toward a professional–family partnership, and using a systems approach to identifying family strengths and needs. Clearly written and well-grounded in current research, *Ordinary Families, Special Children* is enriched by quotes from family members and practitioners.

Shimoni, Rena, Baxter, Joanne, & Kugelmass, Judith. (1992). *Every child is special: Quality group care for infants and toddlers.* Don Mills, Ontario: Addison-Wesley.

This book is a valuable addition to the literature on quality care for infants and toddlers because of its seamless integration of children with special needs into the text and photographs throughout the book. Emphasizing that children with special needs are more like than different from other children, the authors provide practical and specific suggestions for including special needs children in group care. The format of the book is clear, thorough, and useful, with developmental reminders, observation questions, quick tips, and specifics on the role of the caregiver featured throughout the book.

Shore, Rima. (1997). *Rethinking the brain: New insights into early development.* New York: Families and Work Institute.

This beautifully written book presents a clear and engaging overview of recent neuroscientific findings on brain development. Based on the proceedings of a 1996 conference that launched the national "I Am Your Child" Campaign, the book suggests how this research can inform and support efforts to promote the optimal learning and healthy development of young children. The layout, graphics, and beautiful photographs help to make this an attractive and valuable resource for professionals and parents alike.

Silberg, Jackie. (1993). *Games to play with babies.* Beltsville, MD: Gryphon House.
Silberg, Jackie. (1993). *Games to play with toddlers.* Beltsville, MD: Gryphon House.
Silberg, Jackie. (1993). *Games to play with two year olds.* Beltsville, MD: Gryphon House.

These three books are loaded with fun activities for parents and caregivers and their babies, toddlers, and 2-year-olds. With suggested age categories and potential learning identified for each activity, the simple games are clearly described, developmentally appropriate, and incorporate everyday objects found in homes and centers.

Small, Meridith F. (1998). *Our babies, ourselves: How biology and culture shape the way we parent.* New York: Doubleday.

Meridith Small is a professor of antropology at Cornell University and is interested in the interaction of human biology and culture. She begins her book by discussing the new field of "ethnopediatrics," which studies parents and infants across cultures and explores the way different caretaking styles affect the health, well-being, and survival of infants. Focusing especially on the sleeping, crying, and feeding patterns of infants and parents across cultures, she suggests that sleeping with infants, responding immediately to their cries, and feeding on demand or cue are practices better suited to the biology and health of infants than many of our commonly accepted parenting practices. This thought-provoking book is especially recommended for practitioners who work with immigrant families and families who are ethnically diverse.

Smith, Charles A., Cudaback, Dorothea, Goddard, H. Wallace, & Myers-Walls, Judith A. (1994). *National extension parent education model.* Manhattan, KS: Kansas Cooperative Extension Service.

This report is a compilation of priority parent practices and supporting materials to be used as a basis for parent education programming. The authors served as a leadership team for an effort to develop a national parent education model for university-based Extension Services. The model is structured around six roles for parenting: care for self, understand, guide, nurture, motivate, and advocate. Thorough literature reviews are provided for each area. The report offers a wide menu of delivery strategies and concludes with a guide to current parent education curricula.

Sparling, Joseph, Lewis, Isabelle, & Ramey, Craig. (1995). *Partners for learning: Infants, toddlers, and twos (0–36 mos)*. Lewisville, NC: Kaplan.

Used as the curriculum in extensively researched interventions for children aged birth to 3 (the Abecedarian Project and Project CARE), this collection of learning activities is a good resource for child care centers and home visitation programs. It includes an extensive series of adult–child activity cards with cartoons on one side and text on the other side, which may be effectively used by parents with limited reading ability. Supplementing the cards are training guides, handbooks, parent newsletters, and other support materials. The activities and materials emphasize the central role of informational talk rather than directive talk and adult skills such as preparing, attending, modeling, supporting, prompting, rescuing, and building when interacting with very young children. These skills are described in the training portion of the curriculum and enable adults to facilitate rather than impede the natural learning process of young children.

Stonehouse, Anne. (Ed.). (1990). *Trusting toddlers: Planning for one- to three-year-olds in child care centers*. St. Paul, MN: Redleaf Press.

Originally published by the Australian Early Childhood Association, this book is an edited collection of writing by 12 Australian experts in toddler care. As the foreword states, toddlers are a special, wonderful class of people who don't fit into tidy definitions. As such, they often are not well served in group child care. This book celebrates the spontaneous, incredibly curious, wondrous, and often infuriating (to adults) nature of toddlerhood. Its chapters cover toddler characteristics, perspectives on programming, environments, creativity, discipline, routines, play, parent–staff relationships, and staff issues. Its chapter on multicultural programming is full of fresh, practical suggestions. Throughout, *Trusting Toddlers* clarifies the educational potential in everyday caregiving routines. This book is an excellent resource for group care of toddlers and for understanding the psychology of this fascinating age.

Thoman, Evelyn, & Browder, Sue. (1987). *Born dancing: How intuitive parents understand their baby's unspoken language and natural rhythms*. New York: Harper & Row. (out of print)

The first author of this book is a child development researcher, biobehavioral science professor, and mother of six children and four stepchildren. She wrote this book to help parents learn to relax, tune in to their babies, and practice the reciprocal approach to parenting that she calls "danceparenting." Emphasizing the fact that babies are born as individual persons, with a host of personality traits and subtle methods of communication, The authors point out that parents can stop assuming that they are wholly responsible for how their children "turn out." Putting aside this burden of tension and guilt, parents can devote their energies to getting to know their baby as a person and learning the steps of the dance they can enjoy together. After debunking some of what they term, "trivial, inconsequential concerns" common to many parents, the authors discuss the skills and characteristics of normal infants and suggest observation and communication strategies for parents to understand and interact with their babies better. This book would be especially helpful for parents who are tense and overwhelmed by conflicting child-rearing advice or who are concerned that their babies will be less intelligent if they don't learn reading and mathematics before preschool age.

Walsh, David. (1994). *Selling out America's children: How America puts profits before values—and what parents can do.* Minneapolis: Fairview Press.

Written by a psychologist and parent of three children, this book is a wake-up call for today's parents. *Selling Out America's Children* proposes concrete actions parents can take to promote healthy values for their children despite the toxicity of much of our popular culture. Walsh documents our society's emphasis on violence, instant gratification, winning at all costs, rampant consumerism, and individualism at the expense of community. One chapter focuses on the pervasive presence of television, with suggestions for families regarding its constructive use. The author distinguishes between individual and societal responsibility, but argues that our society is exploiting children for profit. Therefore, he suggests that we need to act on changing this society, beginning with our individual families.

Wasik, Barbara H., Bryant, Donna M., & Lyons, Claudia M. (1990). *Home visiting: Procedures for helping families.* Newbury Park, CA: Sage.

Comprehensive, research-based, and practical describe this resource for home visitors and anyone working with home visiting programs, whether from a health, social work, or education background. The authors begin with a historical perspective on home visiting programs in the United States and Europe and follow this with a contemporary philosophical approach to home visiting that is less patronizing and more client centered than some of the earlier home visiting efforts. Issues critical to successful implementation of home visiting are discussed in specific and thorough detail. These include personnel issues, helping skills and techniques, managing and maintaining home visits, stressful situations, ethical and professional issues, and documentation and evaluation in home visiting. Increasingly included today in the menu of helping services for families, home visits can be very effective in serving populations that center-based programs alone may be unable to reach. This book is a valuable tool toward that end.

Weiss, Heather B., & Jacobs, Francine H. (Eds.). (1988). *Evaluating family programs*. Hawthorne, NY: Aldine de Gruyter.

Evaluating family programs is a complex and evolving business, yet it is essential to building credibility and support for these important endeavors. This book is an excellent resource for state-of-the-art evaluation efforts on a wide variety of family support programs. One of its most interesting chapters (by Francine Jacobs) discusses a five-tiered approach to evaluation that clarifies the need for different evaluation goals and strategies at different stages of a program's growth. Too many new programs attempt to assess their outcomes before they take the time for needs and process assessment, essential preliminaries to outcome evaluation. Chapters authored by a raft of evaluation specialists discuss measurement of child, parent, and family outcomes; case studies from the field; and current issues in theory and practice. Two extensive appendices offer a list of research instruments and their sources and a glossary of research and program evaluation terms.

Weissbluth, Marc. (1987). *Healthy sleep habits, happy child*. New York: Ballantine Books.

Of several books on this topic, this is one of the best resources for tired parents. Authored by a researcher and pediatrician who is Director of the Sleep Disorders Center of Chicago's Children's Memorial Hospital, the book begins with an extensive discussion of how children sleep and the importance of healthy sleep habits. Then Dr. Weissbluth systematically discusses the specifics of how parents can help their children establish healthy sleep habits from months 1–4, months 4–12, months 12–36, years 3–6, years 7–12, and in adolescence. Concluding with a chapter on special sleep problems such as sleepwalking and nightmares, and a chapter on special events and concerns such as moving and frequent illnesses, the book is enriched throughout by first-person accounts of parents dealing with their children's sleep problems. The book is refreshingly flexible yet specific in its advice and is developmentally appropriate for the different stages of children's growth.

Williams, Frances. (1996). *Babycare for beginners*. New York: HarperCollins.

Bound in a clever cover that enables the opened book to stand on its own, and generously illustrated throughout with full-color photos that clarify the simple text, this book is a terrific help for new parents and the interventionists and home visitors who work with them. It clearly describes handling your baby, carrying your baby, soothing a crying baby, feeding your baby, diapering, dressing, putting your baby down to sleep, bathing your baby, daily care routines, and signs of illness. The book concludes with a brief section on first aid for babies. A few criticisms are that the photographs of Caucasian families vastly outnumber those of other ethnic groups and that the section on cloth diapering makes the process much more complicated and difficult than it needs to be.

Winer, Michael, & Ray, Karen. (1994). *Collaboration handbook: Creating, sustaining, and enjoying the journey.* St. Paul, MN: Amherst H. Wilder Foundation.

The authors structure their handbook around what they identify as the four stages of collaboration: envision results by working individual to individual, empower ourselves by working individual to organization, ensure success by working organization to organization, and endow continuity by working collaboration to community. Within each of these stages, they provide specific, practical, step-by-step information. Attractively formatted and enriched by case studies and multicultural quotations relating to the collaboration "journey," this book is an excellent resource for anyone planning or setting out on the trip.

Zeanah, Charles H., Jr. (Ed.). (2000, in press). *Handbook of infant mental health* (2nd ed.). New York: Guilford Press.

Zeanah has edited a very comprehensive volume with multiple authors on a spectrum of infant mental health issues. He includes extensive discussions of the context of infant mental health, risk conditions and protective factors, assessment, disorders of infancy, intervention, and social applications of infant mental health. Interdisciplinary in scope, this book is an excellent resource for a wide variety of professionals who work with children from birth to 3 years of age.

RESOURCE GUIDES

The California Department of Education publishes an extensive catalog of educational resources, including their well-known training *Program for Infant/Toddler Caregivers* created with West Ed/Far West Laboratory, which consists of videos, written guides, and trainer's manuals. For information, contact:

California Department of Education
Bureau of Publications, Sales Unit
P.O. Box 271
Sacramento, CA 95812-0271
PH: 916/445-1260

Family Information Services is a helpful resource for parent and family educators. It offers an annual subscription that includes 12 monthly resource packets. The research-based packet materials address family education issues across the life cycle and are developed by experienced family life educators across the country. Materials include presentation guides, handouts, group activities, newsletter articles, book reviews, research updates, and audiotaped interviews with leaders in the field. The materials are photocopy-ready for use in parent education and support groups, workshops, counseling, and organizational newsletters. A Parent and Family Educator's Resource Library of past volumes is also available. For information, contact:

Family Information Services
12565 Jefferson Street NE, Suite 102
Minneapolis, MN 55433
PH: 612/755-6233
TF: 800/852-8112
FX: 612/755-7355
Website: http://www.familyinfoserv.com

Redleaf Press is a nonprofit organization that publishes an annual catalog of quality resources for early childhood professionals. Each item is carefully reviewed before inclusion in the catalog and reflects best thinking in the field. Some of the topical areas are infant and toddler; health, safety, and nutrition; diversity; special needs; guidance and development; child development; training; and family child care. A small number of videos and children's books are included in addition to the extensive collection of books for early childhood professionals. A portion of every purchase contributes to local efforts that support children and families. For information, contact:

Redleaf Press
450 North Syndicate, Suite 5
St. Paul, MN 55104-4125
PH: 651/641-0305
TF: 800/423-8309
FX: 800/641-0115

The *Resource Guide for Early Childhood Family Education* (1994), *Guide for Developing Early Childhood Family Education Programs* (1989), and other helpful curriculum resources are available for purchase through the Minnesota Department of Children, Families and Learning. Many of these resources were authored or compiled by staff of Minnesota's statewide Early Childhood Family Education program, which has combined parent education and early childhood education for Minnesota families of infants, toddlers, and preschoolers since 1974. For further information, contact:

Early Childhood Family Education
Minnesota Department of Children, Families, and Learning
1500 Highway 36 West
Roseville, MN 55113-4266
PH: 651/582-8402
FX: 651/582-8494

Resource Guide: Selected Early Childhood and Early Intervention Training Materials is in its seventh edition (1998) and is an extremely well-organized and comprehensive guide to materials that will be useful for early childhood and intervention preservice and in-service training. Compiled and previewed by Camille Catlett and Pamela Winton of the Frank Porter Graham Child Development Center, the guide is divided into 18 key content areas, with multiple print and audiovisual resources listed for each. Informative annotations are supplied for primary resources, with complete ordering information clearly specified. The publication concludes with a source list of publishers and producers for supplemental resources listed in the guide and two extensive indexes by author and by title. To order, send a $10 check (includes postage and handling) payable to FPG Child Development Center to:

> FPG Child Development Center
> CB#8185
> University of North Carolina
> Chapel Hill, NC 27599-8180
> PH: 919/966-6635

Team Assessment in Early Childhood Special Education: A Trainer's Resource Guide (1988) is edited by Gina Guarneri, Ann Carr, and Linda Brekken of the Infant Preschool Special Education Resource Network of Sacramento, California. Through a federal training grant, this organization developed an intensive 5-day training institute in team assessment of young children with suspected health and developmental needs. This publication is the curriculum for the institute. Its chapter topics include foundations for a family approach to early childhood assessment, development of an assessment team, clinical procedures and interpretations for infant/toddler assessment, observations of the play behavior of infants and young children, foundations for understanding parent–child interaction, cross-cultural issues in assessment, and linking assessment to program planning. Each chapter includes text, training exercises, and an annotated resource bibliography. To order or for further information, contact:

> Resources in Special Education
> 650 Howe Avenue, Suite 300
> Sacramento, CA 95825
> PH: 916/641-5925

ORGANIZATIONS/JOURNALS

The American Academy of Pediatrics publishes a series of informative parent education brochures on a range of health-related infant and toddler topics, with some published in Spanish. Books on caring for infants and children, as well as videotapes on topics such as newborn care and shaken baby syndrome, are also available. For information, contact:

> American Academy of Pediatrics
> Attention: Publications

P.O. Box 747
Elk Grove Village, IL 60007-0747
TF: 800/433-9016
FX: 847/228-1281
Website: http://www.aap.org

The Child and Family Policy Center is a state-based, policy–research implementation organization. It publishes a variety of resources on service integration and on streamlining intake and eligibility services for families. For information, contact:

Child and Family Policy Center
Fleming Building, Suite 102
1218 Sixth Avenue
Des Moines, IA 50309
PH: 515/280-9027
FX: 515/244-8997
E-mail: HN2228@handsnet.org
Website: http://home.earthlink.net/~cfpf/

The Children's Defense Fund (CDF) is a nonprofit research and advocacy organization that exists to provide a voice for American children, especially poor minority children. It attempts to educate the nation about children's needs and encourage preventive investment in this area. The organization publishes a monthly newsletter (*CDF Reports*) geared toward child advocates that provides data and news on federal developments affecting the welfare of children. In addition to the newsletter, CDF publishes many data sources for maternal and child health, child care and development, teen parents, and family income. For information, contact:

Children's Defense Fund Publications
25 E Street NW
Washington, DC 20001
PH: 202/628-8787
TF: 800/CDF-1200
FX: 202/662-3510

The Council for Exceptional Children, Division for Early Childhood (DEC), offers a quarterly publication to its regular and student members called the *Journal of Early Intervention*. Division members also receive quarterly copies of DEC's official newsletter. For information, contact:

CEC Publications
1920 Association Drive
Reston, VA 20191-1589
PH: 703/620-3660
TF: 800/232-7323
FX: 703/264-9494

Early Childhood Research Quarterly reports current research findings on socially and educationally relevant topics. To strengthen the link between research and practice, it includes practitioner commentaries from teachers, program directors, and policymakers. For information, contact:

> Journals Customer Service
> Ablex Publishing Corporation
> 355 Chestnut Street
> Norwood, NJ 07648
> PH: 201/767-8455

Early Education and Development, published quarterly by Psychological Press, Inc., is a cross-disciplinary journal for professionals who serve families and young children from birth to age 8. With a focus on both empirical research and practical application, this highly readable journal is especially useful to early childhood educators, special educators, and researchers in early education and development. For information, contact:

> Subscription Office
> Early Education and Development
> 39 Pearl Street
> Brandon, VT 05733-1007
> PH: 802/247-8312

Family Resource Coalition Report is published quarterly by the Family Resource Coalition of America (FRCA). It usually is organized thematically and aimed at family support workers in the fields of health, education, and social services. It showcases promising programs and practices, and reports on current research relevant to family support programs. FRCA also sponsors a biennial conference and publishes books and reports. For information, contact:

> Family Resource Coalition of America
> 200 South Michigan Avenue, 16th Floor
> Chicago, IL 60604
> PH: 312/341-0900
> FX: 312/341-9361
> E-mail: hn1738@handsnet.org
> Website: http://www.frca.org

Father to Father is an initiative designed to unite fathers with their children and mobilize communities to support fathers and their families. Administered by the Children, Youth, and Family Consortium at the University of Minnesota and overseen by a national board of leaders from the field of father involvement, Father to Father provides resources and technical assistance to organizations and communities that want to support fathers in being a positive force in their children's lives. Available for a nominal charge are "community starter kits" that offer a wide range of ideas and strategies for father involvement, as well as lists of printed materials and resource organizations that can provide professional training. A related website, FatherNet, provides a constantly updated online resource center and discussion groups for fathers and those who care about them. For information, contact:

Father to Father
Children, Youth, and Family Consortium
University of Minnesota
201 Coffey Hall
1420 Eckles Avenue
St. Paul, MN 55108
PH: 612/626-1212
FX: 612/626-1210
Website: http://www.cyfc.umn.edu/FatherNet

Infants and Young Children is an interdisciplinary journal of special care practices published quarterly by Aspen Publishers. Aimed at professionals delivering early intervention and care to at-risk children and children with developmental disabilities, it helps readers deal with the complexities of Pubic Law 99-457 and Public Law 102-119 and stay informed of current research and practice. For subscription information, contact:

Aspen Publishers, Inc.
P.O. Box 990
Frederick, MD 21705-9782
TF: 800/638-8437

Infant Mental Health Journal is the official publication of the World Association for Infant Mental Health (WAIMH). The organization and its publications are dedicated to an interdisciplinary approach to the optimal development of infants and their families. Published four times a year, the journal includes literature reviews, research articles, program descriptions, and book reviews. This is an informative and useful journal for practitioners from varied disciplines. For information, contact:

WAIMH ICYF
Kellogg Center
1 CYF, Suite 1
Michigan State University
East Lansing, MI 48824-1022
PH: 517/432-3793
PH: 212/850-6645 (for journal subscription)
FX: 517/432-3694
Website: http://www.msu.edu/user/waimh

La Leche League International has been dedicated for over 40 years to helping all mothers breastfeed their babies. In addition to their own publications, the organization offers an annotated catalog of resources for parents of infants and toddlers and regional help lines for breastfeeding mothers. For information, contact:

> La Leche League International
> 1400 North Meacham Road
> P.O. Box 4079
> Schaumburg, IL 60173
> PH: 847/519-7730
> PH: 847/519-9585 (Order Department)
> TF: 800/LA-LECHE (Hotline)
> FX: 847/519-7730

MELD is an organization created to support parents by providing easy to understand information in a supportive atmosphere. It provides technical assistance for a wide variety of peer-led parent education programs through publications, curricula, program replication, and training opportunities. For information, contact:

> MELD
> 123 North Third Street, Suite 507
> Minneapolis, MN 55401
> PH: 612/332-7563
> FX: 612/344-1959
> E-mail: MELDctrl@aol.com

Published by and for parents, *Mothering: The Magazine of Natural Family Living* is an alternative to many parent magazines found on newsstands. Its views on vaccination, circumcision, infant sleep patterns, breastfeeding, and other issues are likely to be different from those found in mainstream magazines and are not for everyone. *Mothering*'s emphasis on the importance and value of parenting and on the needs and rights of children is consistent, however, and refreshing. For information, contact:

> *Mothering* Magazine, Inc.
> P.O. Box 1690
> Santa Fe, NM 87504
> TF: 800/984-8116
> FX: 505/986-8335
> E-mail: @mothering.com
> Website: http://www.mothering.com

Prevent Child Abuse America has a broad collection of simply written pamphlets and brochures to assist parents in caring for their children. The organization works to expand and disseminate knowledge about child abuse prevention and promote sound policy development and prevention programs. For information, contact:

Prevent Child Abuse America
200 South Michigan Avenue, 17th Floor
Chicago, IL 60604
PH: 312/663-3520
TF: 800/835-2671 (publications only)
FX: 312/939-8962
E-mail: ncpca@childabuse.org
Website: http://www.childabuse.org

The National Council on Family Relations (NCFR) has a catalog of scholarly publications on families and publishes two quarterly journals: *Journal of Marriage and the Family* and *Family Relations: Journal of Applied Family and Child Studies*. NCFR also hosts an annual conference. For information, contact:

National Council on Family Relations
3989 Central Avenue NE, Suite 550
Minneapolis, MN 55421
PH: 612/781-9331
TF: 888/781-9331
FX: 612/781-9348
E-mail: ncfr3989@ncfr.com
Website: http://www.ncfr.com

The National Indian Child Welfare Association (NICWA) focuses on community development efforts, public policy development, and information exchange related to the welfare of Native American children and their families. It provides cultural competency training to help organizations develop this trait throughout their policies, procedures, practices, and values. NICWA also produces publications and provides other technical assistance. For information, contact:

National Indian Child Welfare Association
3611 SW Hood Street, Suite 201
Portland, OR 97201
PH: 503/222-4044
FX: 503/222-4007
E-mail: info@nicwa.org

The National Organization for Rare Disorders (NORD) was created by and for people concerned about "orphan diseases," defined as rare, debilitating illnesses that strike small numbers of people. The central goals of the organization are to promote scientific research on the cause, treatment, and cure of rare disorders; educate the general public and medical profession about same; and act as a clearinghouse for information about rare disorders and for linking families with similar disorders together for mutual support. For information, contact:

National Organization for Rare Disorders
100 Route 37

P.O. Box 8923
New Fairfield, CT 06812-1783
PH: 203/746-6518
TF: 800/999-6673
FX: 203/746-6481
E-mail: orphan@nord-rdb.com
Website: http:/www.NORD-RDB.com/~orphan

The PACER Center is a nonprofit organization that serves families of children and young adults with disabilities. Staffed primarily by parents of youth with disabilities, PACER provides workshops, individual assistance, and written information on legislation and services relating to individuals with physical, mental, learning, or emotional disabilities. PACER publishes two free newsletters and has produced a disability awareness puppet program and dozens of booklets, handouts, videotapes, training manuals, workshop outlines, and transparencies. For further information, contact:

PACER Center, Inc.
4826 Chicago Avenue South
Minneapolis, MN 55417-1098
PH: 612/827-2966
PH: 612/827-7770 (TTY)
TF: 800/537-2237 (Minnesota only)
E-mail: pacer@pacer.org
Website: http://www.pacer.org

As its title implies, *Topics in Early Childhood Special Education* is a quarterly journal featuring research-based articles on current issues in the field. For information, contact:

PRO-ED Journals
8700 Shoal Creek Boulevard
Austin, TX 78757-6897
PH: 512/451-3246

Young Children, published six times a year by the National Association for the Education of Young Children (NAEYC), is aimed at readers who work with young children from birth through age 8. It provides a scholarly, yet readable approach to research and theory and how they relate to good classroom practice. NAEYC sponsors an annual conference and publishes a variety of books, brochures, videos, and posters on early childhood topics. The organization is the originator and publisher of the recently revised *Developmentally Appropriate Practice in Early Childhood Programs*. For information, contact:

NAEYC
1509 16th Street NW

Washington, DC 20036-1426
PH: 202/232-8777
TF: 800/424-2460
FX: 202/328-1846
E-mail: membership@naeyc.org
Website: http://www.naeyc.org

The *Zero to Three* bulletin, published bimonthly by the National Center for Infants, Toddlers, and Families, is aimed at professionals working with both typical and special needs infants and toddlers in a variety of settings. Scholarly and clinical in style, *Zero to Three* keeps health, education, and social service professionals abreast of the current research and practice pertinent to infants and toddlers. The Zero to Three Center also sponsors an annual training institute and award-winning website for parents and practitioners. It publishes excellent books and reports on infant and toddler issues. For information, contact:

Zero to Three
National Center for Infants, Toddlers, and Families
734 15th Street NW, Suite 1000
Washington, DC 20005-1013
PH: 202/638-1144
TF: 800/899-4301 (orders only)
FX: 202/638-0851
E-mail: 0to3@zerotothree.org
Website: http://www.zerotothree.org

VIDEOS

Child Development Media, Inc. is an extensive collection of over 300 videotapes and other resources for early intervention, early education, and general child development. Some of the many topic areas included are assessment and planning, children in groups, child development from birth through adolescence, health and disability issues, language and communication, parenting, and staff development. Each item in the catalog has been previewed and represents current thinking and best practice in the field. According to the catalog, every purchase from Child Development Media, Inc. funds either direct service for children and families or the production of new materials. For information, contact;

Child Development Media, Inc.
5632 Van Nuys Boulevard, Suite 286
Van Nuys, CA 91401
PH: 818/994-0933
TF: 800/405-8942
FX: 818/994-0153

The First Three Years: A Guide to Selected Videos for Parents and Professionals was designed and published collaboratively by three national organizations. It reviews more than 50 videos chosen by child development experts and targeted toward a general audience of parents and professionals. Each review includes a summary of the video's contents, suggested audience, supplemental materials, language, and length, as well as information for ordering. To order a free copy of the video guide, call 888/777-2744 or 212/606-3840. The full text of the guide is also available online at http://www.cmwf.org.

The First Years Last Forever is a 30-minute video describing the vital importance of parenting and caregiving in the first months and years of life. Produced by the "I am Your Child" campaign, it is available for $5 to cover postage and handling from Johnson & Johnson. Call 888/447-3400 to order a copy.

Seeing Is Believing is a 40-minute video, with accompanying instructional manual, designed to introduce home visitors to a strength-focused strategy for videotaping parents and infants and then viewing the tape together in a spirit of shared discovery and self-reflection. Produced in 1999 by the University of Minnesota, in cooperation with the Minnesota Department of Children, Families and Learning and the Minnesota Department of Health, the video and manual are currently available. For information, contact:

> Irving B. Harris Training Center for Infant and Toddler Development
> Institute for Child Development
> 196 Child Development
> 51 East River Road
> University of Minnesota
> Minneapolis, MN 55455-0345
> PH: 612/624-4510
> FX: 612/624-6373

Ten Things Every Child Needs is a 60-minute documentary produced by Chicago public television and funded by a local Chicago foundation. Highly recommended by the NAEYC, it discusses how children's early experiences from birth on influence brain development and shape their ability to learn. The 10 simple things it describes to help children develop are interaction; loving touch; stable relationships; safe, healthy environments; self-esteem; quality child care; play; communication; music; and reading. To obtain a copy, send $10 (check or money order) to:

> Robert R. McCormick Tribune Foundation
> Attention: Ten Things
> 435 North Michigan Avenue, Suite 770
> Chicago, IL 60611

Index

("t" indicates a table)